To Improve Health and Health Care
1997

Stephen L. Isaacs and
James R. Knickman, Editors

Foreword by Steven A. Schroeder

To Improve Health and Health Care *1997*

The Robert Wood Johnson Foundation Anthology

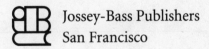 Jossey-Bass Publishers
San Francisco

Substantial discounts on bulk quantities of Jossey-Bass books are available to corporations, professional associations, and other organizations. For details and discount information, contact the special sales department at Jossey-Bass Inc., Publishers (415) 433-1740; Fax (800) 605-2665.

For sales outside the United States, please contact your local Simon & Schuster International Office.

Jossey-Bass Web address: http://www.josseybass.com

 Manufactured in the United States of America on Lyons Falls Turin Book. This paper is acid-free and 100 percent totally chlorine-free.

Library of Congress Cataloging-in-Publication Data

To improve health and health care, 1997: the Robert Wood Johnson Foundation
    anthology / Stephen L. Isaacs and James R. Knickman, editors.
    — 1st ed.
        p.   cm.
    Includes index.
    ISBN 0-7879-0909-2 (alk. paper)
    1. Public health—Research grants—United States.   2. Public
health—United States—Endowments.   3. Robert Wood Johnson
Foundation.   I. Isaacs, Stephen L.   II. Knickman, James.
III. Robert Wood Johnson Foundation.
    [DNLM: 1. Delivery of Health Care—United States.   W 84 AA1 T5
1997]
RA440.87.U6T6   1997
610'.79'73—dc21
DNLM/DLC
for Library of Congress   97-16892

FIRST EDITION
PB Printing   10 9 8 7 6 5 4 3 2 1

Contents

—ᴡᴡ— Foreword

Foundations dedicated to remedying social ills face a particular challenge: how to communicate to the public the rationale for and results of the programs that they fund. The Robert Wood Johnson Foundation, like other foundations in the public eye, gets the word out through avenues such as annual reports, newsletters, monographs, news releases, the World Wide Web, and conference presentations.

With the publication of *To Improve Health and Health Care, 1997: The Robert Wood Johnson Foundation Anthology,* we are attempting to share information in a new way. In *To Improve Health and Health Care, 1997,* the people most familiar with a selection of our programs—their evaluators and directors in most cases—discuss the reasons the programs were undertaken, examine what happened as they were implemented, and explore lessons that can be learned from them. Written clearly and, we hope, without jargon, the book is intended to reach not only our traditional audience of public policy professionals but also a wider audience consisting of other foundations' officers and trustees and members of the public interested in health and health care.

While the authors do not speak for the Foundation, they offer insights about our values—values expressed through the programs we felt were important enough to fund. These values are best captured by the statement of our mission, "to improve the health and health care of all Americans," and by the strategies the Foundation has adopted to fulfill that mission: increasing access to basic health care for Americans of all ages, improving services for people with chronic illnesses, and reducing the harm caused by substance abuse.

Although the chapters selected for this volume present only a sample of the Foundation's activities, they offer a glimpse of the richness and diversity of our interests. A more complete picture will emerge with the publication of future volumes of the anthology over the coming years.

To Improve Health and Health Care, 1997 opens our philosophical and programmatic books to public scrutiny. It attempts to demystify what the Foundation does and to let the public in on the programs it funds, why it funds them, and what it has learned from its successes and failures. The publication offers the hope that we can learn from the past and not, as philosopher George Santayana feared, be condemned to repeat it.

Princeton, New Jersey   STEVEN A. SCHROEDER, M.D.
May 1997   President
                                                        The Robert Wood Johnson Foundation

—ww— **Introduction**

When Gen. Robert Wood Johnson, the former chairman of Johnson & Johnson and head of Franklin D. Roosevelt's effort to mobilize small business in support of the war effort, died, in 1968, he left the bulk of his billion-dollar estate to a small foundation bearing his name. At that time, The Robert Wood Johnson Foundation gave grants within the state of New Jersey, primarily in the New Brunswick area. When the estate was settled, in 1972, The Robert Wood Johnson Foundation was transformed into a major national philanthropy. Today, with assets of more than $5 billion, it is one of the nation's largest foundations.

Describing the mission of the Foundation is deceptively simple: to improve the health and health care of all Americans. To fulfill that mission, the Foundation provides grants that further one of three goals articulated in 1991:

1. *Increasing access to basic health care for Americans of all ages.*
   From its earliest days, the Foundation zeroed in on access, particularly access to primary care. Initially, this emphasis was based on the assumption (an incorrect one, as it turned out) that national health insurance was just around the corner and that the supply of primary health services would not meet the demand that health care reform would generate. Early grants focused on expanding the availability of emergency medical services, developing perinatal care networks, and increasing the supply of generalist physicians and other health practitioners.

   In the 1980s and 1990s, the Foundation emphasized access for underserved and vulnerable populations, such as residents of inner cities and rural areas, minorities, individuals with chronic illnesses, and indigent and uninsured individuals. It launched programs to encourage minorities to become physicians, as well as demonstrations to show innovative ways of providing services.

Current initiatives directed to improving access to health care include grants to encourage reform efforts that expand health insurance coverage, support of local efforts encouraging practicing physicians to volunteer their services to needy individuals, and establishment of a center tracking how the changing health care markets in sixty communities affect the health and health care of local residents.

2. *Improving services for people with chronic illnesses.* The Foundation's concern about chronic illness dates back at least to 1982, when it announced a goal of helping people maintain or regain maximum attainable function in their daily lives. Beginning in 1988, the Foundation targeted medical and social systems of care for people with specific chronic illnesses. Since then, a series of grants has provided support to local agencies and communities to experiment with ideas to better coordinate services for people with chronic illnesses. The Foundation has financed initiatives such as the On Lok program in San Francisco and its successors, which provided funding to single agencies offering the full range of services needed by frail elderly persons and others with chronic conditions.

   Currently, the Foundation is in the process of awarding grants to eight hundred interfaith religious coalitions to create programs encouraging volunteers to assist chronically ill members of their communities. Additionally, grant programs are attempting to improve services to individuals at the end of life and to develop better service systems under managed care for people with chronic conditions. On the analysis side, the Foundation has studies aimed at better understanding the needs of the chronically ill and has published *Chronic Care in America,* a chartbook outlining the dimensions of chronic illness in America and the challenges facing people with chronic conditions.[1]

3. *Reducing the harm caused by substance abuse.* The Foundation's mission has always emphasized improvement of *health* and health care. However, the Foundation's targeting of substance abuse as a key concern in 1991 was the first time it had given such high priority to an area largely outside traditional health care services. In support of this goal, the Foundation

has focused primarily on strategies to reduce demand for tobacco, alcohol, and illicit drugs. A flagship initiative, the Fighting Back Program, has supported community-based endeavors in fourteen communities that bring together local forces attempting to reduce substance abuse.

The Foundation has given special attention to keeping young people from beginning to smoke, drink, or use illicit substances. A $20 million grant was recently awarded to the Center for Tobacco-Free Kids to make the public more aware of the importance of curtailing the availability of tobacco products for young people. The Smokeless States Initiative funds statewide coalitions to reduce access to tobacco products. A peer-reviewed, investigator-initiated grant program is funding research on how public policy could better combat the damage caused by substance abuse.

In 1996, the Foundation awarded a total of $267 million in support of programs to advance these three goals. Twenty-eight percent ($76 million) of the funds were for programs to advance the Foundation's access goal, 14 percent ($38 million) to advance its chronic care goal, and 39 percent ($103 million) to advance its substance-abuse goal. In addition, it awarded $36 million for programs aimed at finding ways to contain the rising cost of health care, a topic that has also been of importance to the Foundation, and $14 million for other programs, primarily ones carried out in the New Brunswick, New Jersey, area.

Another way to describe what the Foundation does is to look at the strategies used in furthering its goals. In 1996, 31 percent of its grant funds were awarded for demonstration projects, 15 percent for education and training, 24 percent for research and policy analysis, and 20 percent to communications. The remaining 10 percent went to evaluations, conferences, technical assistance, and other programmatic uses.

Although the Foundation's resources are clearly substantial, they must be placed in the context of a nation that spends more than a *trillion* dollars annually on health care. Given the relatively small contribution of the Foundation, its ability to improve health and health care depends on the strength of the ideas it funds, the quality of its programs and grantees, and the ability to learn from the experiences of its grantees and transmit this information widely.

The Foundation therefore places great emphasis on evaluating its major national programs and having results reported in journal articles, monographs, newsletters, audiovisual materials, and conference presentations.

To Improve Health and Health Care, 1997 builds on the Foundation's traditional means of sharing information and goes beyond them. It provides an in-depth look at some of the Foundation's programs—warts and all—by those who know them best. It is intended to complement the Foundation's *Annual Report* and its newsletter, *Advances*, by offering a deeper analysis that is, we hope, more readable than most journal articles.

It is not, however, a substitute for the detailed presentation of findings about specific programs that have, in many cases, been published in academic journals. The journal articles cited in this book are mainly directed at the specialist with an interest in a given area. By contrast, *To Improve Health and Health Care, 1997* focuses more on informed assessments of the Foundation's strategies and on the larger lessons learned from the programs presented in these pages.

In any single volume, we can examine only a small sample of the Foundation's work. In 1996 alone, it funded 870 different programs, and over two thousand grants were active. Choices had to be made about which programs to present in this book. The chapter subjects were selected on the basis of whether a recent evaluation had been done, whether a program was sufficiently far along to merit inclusion, and whether the findings would advance knowledge in the field.

To Improve Health and Health Care, 1997 is organized around three major subject areas: access to health care services, the changing health care system, and the Foundation's efforts to improve services for vulnerable groups. In many cases, these categories intertwine with one another. For example, a study of services for disabled people in Springfield, Massachusetts, ultimately has to do with the first two subject areas, access to care and how care is affected by changes in the system.

ACCESS TO HEALTH CARE SERVICES

The first three chapters concern access to health care services. In Chapter One, "Reach Out: Physicians' Initiative to Expand Care to Underserved Americans," the program's evaluator, journalist Irene Wielawski, chronicles how committed physicians from Tallahassee to

Sacramento have mobilized their colleagues on behalf of the uninsured. She observes that, ironically, this is happening just as the commercialization of the health care system is dampening the spirit of volunteerism the program seeks to channel.

As one way of increasing access to health care services, the Foundation funded programs to improve the health care workforce. In Chapter Two, "Improving the Health Care Workforce: Perspectives from Twenty-Four Years' Experience," the Foundation's president, Steven Schroeder, its executive vice president, Lewis Sandy, and an outside analyst, Stephen Isaacs, examine the Foundation's workforce efforts over nearly a quarter century. They cite both successes and failures; based on the experiences to date, they offer guidance for future workforce programs.

Much of what we know about access to care comes from four Foundation-funded surveys conducted between 1976 and 1994. These surveys build a solid base of reliable information upon which policy makers can act. In the third chapter, "A Review of the National Access-to-Care Surveys," Project HOPE policy analysts Marc Berk and Claudia Schur offer an inside perspective first on how researchers met some of the methodological challenges in conducting these surveys and second on the substance of the surveys and their importance for public policy.

THE CHANGING HEALTH CARE SYSTEM

As the three chapters in the second section make clear, access to care is affected by changes in the health care system—particularly the sweep of managed care, the rise of for-profit health systems, increased concern with cost containment, and the shift of services from the federal to state governments. To gain a better understanding of the system and to try to improve it, the Foundation supported a number of initiatives, three of which are examined here.

In Chapter Four, "Expertise Meets Politics: Efforts to Work with States," Beth Stevens, Foundation senior program officer, and Prof. Lawrence Brown of Columbia University discuss lessons from a national program that provided grants to states to test different models of health care reform. The authors stress that foundations, which view their work as apolitical, must always be aware that policy change is ultimately influenced by politics and is likely to stir local rivalries, engender conflicts, and become messy and partisan.

In Chapter Five, "The Media and Change in Health Systems," Marc Kaplan, senior communications officer at the Foundation, and Mark Goldberg, distinguished fellow at the Yale University School of Management, report on a series of media briefings they organized to help journalists understand the changing health care system. Given the importance of the media, the authors conclude with a series of tips on how health professionals can better explain to journalists the forces now driving health care.

One of the most dramatic of these forces is the drive to reduce costs, or at least slow their rate of increase. In the 1980s and early 1990s, the public perception was that malpractice lawsuits resulting in excessive awards by easily swayed juries were driving physicians out of medical practice and adding billions to the nation's health care bill. Through a series of grants, the Foundation sought to discover the gravity of the malpractice situation, investigate its root causes, and explore alternatives for resolving disputes between patients and physicians. The results are summarized in Chapter Six, "Addressing the Problem of Medical Malpractice," by health policy analyst Joel Cantor and his colleagues.

VULNERABLE POPULATIONS

The changing health care system and the political policies jeopardizing the safety net pose a threat to the nation's most vulnerable populations, who are the subject of the final section of the book. While The Robert Wood Johnson Foundation strives to improve the health and health care of *all* Americans, it has devoted greatest attention to those who are especially vulnerable: individuals who are disabled, indigent, and uninsured; seniors; children; and people with AIDS.

In Springfield, Massachusetts, Brown University professors Susan Allen and Vincent Mor surveyed the health and social services available to disabled adults. Chapter Seven, "Unmet Need in the Community: The Springfield Study," describes an all-too-typical situation where services are characterized by gaps, limitations, lack of continuity, and poor coordination. Finding that many disabled people lack services and money to meet anything more than their basic needs, the authors conclude that "the status quo doesn't work."

SUPPORT (an acronym for Study to Understand Prognoses and Preferences for Outcomes and Risks of Treatments) was a multiyear project that examined how decisions were made by and for gravely ill, hospitalized patients facing death. The results of the study—especially the finding that physicians did not understand patients' preferences—were widely reported in the media. In Chapter Eight, "Unexpected Returns: Insights from SUPPORT," George Washington University professor Joanne Lynn, who codirected the study, reflects upon the ramifications of the largest study of dying people ever conducted in this country.

The Foundation has consistently supported programs designed to improve children's health. One program, All Kids Count, is now a collaborative effort with four other foundations and the U.S. Centers for Disease Control and Prevention to develop systems to track immunizations of preschool children. In Chapter Nine, "Developing Child Immunization Registries: The All Kids Count Program," University of North Carolina health systems analyst Gordon DeFriese and his colleagues share early results of an evaluation of this program. They discuss the constraints to maintaining computerized immunization registries and offer suggestions to a nation poised to develop extensive state and local immunization registry systems.

In 1990, the Foundation, in collaboration with the U.S. Department of Housing and Urban Development, launched a nine-city demonstration project to help homeless families obtain HUD-supported housing and find social services. In Chapter Ten, "The Homeless Families Program: A Summary of Key Findings," Vanderbilt University health policy researcher Debra Rog and Foundation senior program officer Marjorie Gutman explain how the complexity and fragmentation of service systems, combined with the many deeply rooted needs of homeless families, hamper efforts such as these to bring about true change.

The AIDS epidemic justified research outside of the normal purview of the Foundation: a survey of Americans' sexual behavior and practices. Promised federal government funding for the study was withdrawn because the research was viewed as too controversial. Robert Michael of the University of Chicago and his colleagues then approached the Foundation, which became the first of several foundations to fund this groundbreaking research. The National Health and Social Life Survey received national media attention and was the basis for two books and many scholarly articles. In the final chapter, "The National Health and Social Life Survey: Public Health Findings and Their Implications," the survey's codirector, Robert Michael, pulls together the public health implications of the survey.

As managed care and commercial enterprise continue to transform health care; government budgets for social services are reduced; an aging population suffers more from chronic than acute illnesses; and unhealthy behaviors, including substance abuse, create serious social and medical problems, those concerned with health and health care face important challenges. *To Improve Health and Health Care, 1997* recounts how one foundation is attempting to meet these challenges. We hope that it proves useful to those working to improve the health care system as well as those trying to understand and navigate it.

Princeton, New Jersey   STEPHEN L. ISAACS
May 1997   JAMES R. KNICKMAN

Endnote

1. C. Hoffman and D. Rice, *Chronic Care in America: A 21st Century Challenge* (Princeton, N.J.: The Robert Wood Johnson Foundation, 1996).

⟨⟨⟨ Acknowledgments

This book reflects the dedication and thoughtfulness of a great many people, to whom we would like to express our gratitude.

Within The Robert Wood Johnson Foundation, Frank Karel, vice president for communications, provided vision, guidance, and sound judgment from the beginning. His contribution to the book is significant and appreciated. Lewis Sandy, Steven Schroeder, and Vicki Weisfeld read the chapters in draft and offered important suggestions for improving them. Linda Potts, Deborah Malloy, and Sherry Georgianna provided invaluable administrative and clerical services.

An outside committee consisting of William Morrill, Patricia Patrizi, and Jonathan Showstack reviewed each manuscript for objectivity and lack of bias. Their fairness and toughness added immeasurably to the quality of the book. C. P. Crow, a longtime editor at *The New Yorker,* served as the book's editor. His contributions to the style and clarity of the final product cannot be overestimated. Molly McKaughan did a last-minute, and much appreciated, review of the next-to-last draft.

Special thanks are owed to our research and editorial assistant, Dilshad Shahid, who worked tirelessly and with good humor on the various tasks, many of them unglamorous, that transform an idea into a printed work. At Family Care International, Jill Sheffield and Caryn Levitt handled grant management and financial reporting requirements rapidly and effectively.

Finally, we would like to thank the chapter authors for the care that they gave to this endeavor and for the high quality of their work.

S.L.I.
J.R.K.

—⟋⟍⟍— Reach Out
Physicians' Initiative
to Expand Care to
Underserved Americans

Irene M. Wielawski

Editors' Introduction

To increase the availability of health services to all Americans, all parts of society need to expand their efforts and responsibilities. Government programs are part of the solution; individuals play key roles; and the voluntary efforts of neighbors, providers, and community institutions are crucial. The Robert Wood Johnson Foundation has supported a range of efforts over the years to encourage this breadth of voluntarism.

Chapter One reports on the early experiences of Reach Out, a program to encourage volunteer services from the physician community. Other Foundation programs to encourage voluntarism include Faith in Action, which provides startup funding for approximately eight hundred faith-based organizations of volunteers that extend support services to the chronically ill, and the Service Credit Banking program, which encourages healthy seniors to care for frail members of their communities. The volunteers receive service credits that can be redeemed as they themselves age and require support services.

Reach Out encourages locally based groups of physicians to design innovative approaches that expand primary care services for people who lack health insurance and the ability to pay for medical care. This chapter explains how the program works, describes some of the innovations that have been implemented, and outlines the complexity of doing volunteer work in the emerging world of market-driven health care.

Irene M. Wielawski was charged with doing an evaluation of the project, but she is far from the standard evaluator. Before accepting the Reach Out assignment, she was an investigative reporter for the *Los Angeles Times*. Rather than using traditional social science evaluation methods for this project, the Foundation decided that an investigative reporter was best equipped to sort through the experiences and draw lessons that might emerge from them. Narrowly defined access outcomes are of less interest in this evaluation than are the defining qualitative stories and lessons about how to encourage volunteerism. Physicians historically have provided large amounts of charity care to needy patients; the challenge considered herein is how this commitment can be translated to the 1990s medical care environment.

In the autumn of 1993, the nation's 550,000 private practicing physicians were challenged to take up the cause of people who had poor access to medical care. Behind the idea was the recognition that a large gap existed between the health care capacity those physicians represented and the actual number of people benefiting from their skills. A lack of insurance, the wrong kind of insurance, geography, location, economics, prejudice, language—all were factors separating the doctors from the needy patients. If a significant number of doctors in private practice could be mobilized to use their knowledge of the health care system on behalf of excluded patients, real progress might be made in improving access. At the same time, a badly demoralized profession might find its way back to the basic principles of altruism and social responsibility—the underpinnings of the medical profession.

It was an interesting idea for interesting times. President Bill Clinton, elected the previous November partly on a promise of overhauling the nation's patchwork system of health care, was putting the finishing touches on his comprehensive reform plan. Congress was studying other proposals. All of the proposals emphasized finding a means of payment as the way to accomplish universal access to health care. Some featured a Canadian-style government-run system, others focused on correcting inequities in the insurance market. Health reform was front-page news, and polls showed overwhelming popular support for it.

Of course, many insurance-related issues were still unsettled. Was a single payer system preferable? Should the government run it? What was the role of employers? Did anyone have a reliable cost estimate? Nevertheless, it seemed certain that government would do something for Americans without health insurance, whose numbers at that time were estimated at thirty-seven million.

Into this maelstrom sailed The Robert Wood Johnson Foundation with a $12 million, five-year program called Reach Out: Physicians' Initiative to Expand Care to Underserved Americans. Launched in September 1993, the program has encountered rough water ever since, tossed like every other player in health care by the political and economic turbulence of the 1990s: the failure of national reform, the bruising marketplace free-for-all that followed, the rise of managed care, and, more recently, uncertain signals from Washington about the future of Medicaid and Medicare. Despite the odds, thirty-nine out of forty Reach Out projects have survived, and some have proved remarkably nimble at using their small size and relatively loose structures to take advantage of opportunities presented by change.

The projects have also illustrated the portability of late House Speaker Thomas P. "Tip" O'Neill's oft-quoted wisdom that "all politics is local." Poor health and expensive crisis care may be the result of inadequate access to medical services, whether one is a non-English-speaking immigrant in East Los Angeles or a ranch hand in rural Montana. But the barriers to access are often uniquely local and not entirely defined by a lack of insurance—the issue that garnered most of the attention during the two-year debate on health reform. Indeed, the giant-sized mock-up of a Health Security Card, unveiled by President Clinton at a press conference in 1993 and reproduced in newspapers and magazines around the country, was a clever bit of marketing that came to symbolize the solution for millions of working, uninsured Americans who could not pay their medical bills. Yet many worse-off citizens who were already enrolled in the government's Medicaid program could testify to the empty promise of an insurance card in places where doctors, hospitals, testing labs, and pharmacies rejected it, or where other circumstances of poverty—lack of a car, for instance—made it impossible to obtain medical care.

The Reach Out site in Dillon, Montana, is wrestling with some of these local factors. The community's twenty-two-bed hospital and handful of physicians serve sparsely populated Beaverhead County. The county covers rugged terrain along the Continental Divide in the southwestern corner of Montana, an area roughly equivalent in size to Connecticut and Rhode Island but with fewer than ten thousand residents. A central question for the project is how to get people to come in for early, cost-effective treatment. The seasonal demands of ranching and the absence of public transportation make routine trips to the doctor inconvenient, at best. Also, ranchers are far more likely to provide bunks and meals than health insurance for their workers.

Contrast the challenges in Montana with those faced by two projects in Los Angeles trying to augment the capacity of overwhelmed public agencies through partnerships with the city's abundant supply of private physicians and hospitals. On paper, it looks simple, a win-win situation for everyone—most of all needy patients. But the key partner here, the Los Angeles County Department of Health Services,

is in turmoil, a victim of California's deep recession, antiquated facilities, and shortsighted management. The headlines in the last few years
have focused not on patients but on the latest budget crisis or administrative overhaul. Besides the instability of their major partner, the
projects must contend with the sheer volume of need in Los Angeles
County, where by some estimates 2.7 million people lack health insurance. One project, headed by a pediatrician, Neal D. Kaufman, is trying to recruit physicians in private practice to help care for children
in Los Angeles County's vast foster care system. Kaufman's goal is to
assign each child to a network of trained pediatricians, so that even if
the foster home changes, as it frequently does, the medical care
remains consistently in the hands of physicians familiar with the special needs of foster children, and each child's medical history. But the
project is contending with a county caseload that averages seventy-
three thousand children at any one time and shifts by about fifteen
thousand each month as children are reunited with families, are
adopted, or otherwise leave the system, according to Elena Halpert-
Schilts, the project manager. "We are trying to put together a small
pilot effort and hope that it works well enough to become a model for
the larger system," she said.

It is too soon to measure Reach Out's collective impact on health
care access, and impossible to predict whether these community-based
experiments will carry sufficient momentum nationally to significantly
lessen hardships faced by underserved Americans. Indeed, estimates
of the uninsured are creeping ever upward, totaling some forty-one
million in 1996—four million more than when Reach Out began.
Some projects, though, are clearly succeeding in keeping the needs of
the underserved on the radar screen, no small accomplishment in these
profit-driven times when mergers, acquisitions, and price-earnings
ratios dominate the conversation in health care circles.

HOW REACH OUT WORKS

Reach Out has thirty-nine sites in twenty-four states and the District
of Columbia. They are provided with direction and technical support
by a national program office based at the Brown University Center for
Primary Care and Prevention in Pawtucket, Rhode Island. The office
is headed by H. Denman Scott, an internist who is associate dean at
Brown University School of Medicine. Its deputy director is Melinda L.
Thomas, who comes from a health policy and planning background.

Chaired by James G. Nuckolls, a rural physician from Galax, Virginia, a fourteen-member national advisory committee assisted in choosing the grantees from two separate applicant pools and continues to advise the project. In the first application round, 244 proposals were received and 22 were selected for funding in August 1994. A second call for proposals yielded 194 more applicants; of these, 18 were chosen in August 1995. Each successful applicant received a one-year planning grant of up to $100,000, and each was eligible for three-year implementation grants of up to $200,000, with eligibility based on a readiness to carry out goals formulated in the planning year. None of the money can be used to pay for the treatment of underserved patients. This restriction encourages grantees to reorganize their communities' existing resources into a system from which greater numbers can benefit. Grantees are expected to find permanent, local funding after four years of Robert Wood Johnson Foundation support.

What is a typical Reach Out project? There isn't one, largely because of the variability in local conditions illustrated by the Montana and Los Angeles examples. The design of each project was also left to the physician leaders and their local partners, in the belief that they best knew their community's needs and how physicians might be used to alleviate those needs. The result is a smorgasbord of approaches, with certain conceptual similarities.

The majority of the Reach Out projects rely on a cadre of volunteer physicians, but some projects use a free-clinic approach while others strive to integrate underserved patients directly into the practices of participating physicians. Not all projects define the underserved as uninsured. In Montgomery, Alabama, for example, the Child Health Access Project is trying to increase the number of private pediatricians willing to see children insured by Medicaid. The project, headed by Robert Beshear and A. Z. Holloway, Jr., both pediatricians, is building on a successful obstetrical access project and seeks to remedy a situation in which more than half of the low-income and Medicaid-insured babies born in a four-county area do not receive recommended pediatric screenings and timely immunizations. The majority of these children have no access to regular pediatric care and must rely instead on bare-bones public clinics and hospital emergency rooms for crisis care.

The Montgomery project so far has succeeded in doubling the number of private pediatricians who accept Medicaid-insured children into their practices. But its greater accomplishment over time may be in breaking down long-standing attitudinal barriers to serving these children. Because of a shortage of pediatricians in greater Montgomery, those in private practice have found it relatively easy to claim high caseload as an excuse for excluding poor children. The underlying reasons, however, are more insidious: deep-seated mistrust and confusion about the state's Medicaid program, and a private-practice medical culture that has seen poor children as primarily the responsibility of public agencies. This scenario is more typical than not in Reach Out projects. The hope is that these negative attitudes, like other forms of prejudice, will moderate, in this case through new exposure to Medicaid-insured youngsters and their parents, better education about the state's Medicaid program, and case management provided by the Reach Out staff.

Case management is seen by Beshear and Holloway as critical to the project's success, so that low-income patients with problems that exceed the resources of a pediatrician's office—transportation, child care, social service needs, for example—are linked up with appropriate community services.

Some Reach Out projects are statewide efforts. In South Carolina, a project led by Charleston neurosurgeon Bartolo M. Barone has greatly simplified the bureaucratic process of obtaining drugs from the charity programs of pharmaceutical manufacturers, making it possible for needy patients to get prescriptions filled free at their local pharmacies.

Other Reach Out projects are much more local, targeting a special population in a single municipality. In Louisville, Kentucky, for example, the Reach Out effort, headed by two internists, Mary A. Henry and Will W. Ward, Jr., has helped bring volunteer medical services to shelters for the homeless, recovering drug addicts, and alcoholics. Some urban Reach Out projects are working with new immigrants and others for whom language and culture form significant barriers to care. Other projects are in rural areas, where distance, geography, and a dearth of physicians limit access. Some projects, notably the seven in California, are operating in markets saturated by managed care. Others are in areas where the majority of physicians are still practicing fee-for-service medicine.

Finally, not all Reach Out projects are primary-care models. In San Francisco—a city with an enviable network of volunteer and county-run clinics and a large, full-service public hospital—surgeon William P. Schecter's Reach Out project runs a free Saturday-morning surgery program for uninsured people with hernias or other minor problems that can be treated on an outpatient basis. Because their conditions are not life threatening, these patients fall through the cracks even in a comprehensive public health care system like San Francisco's.

Another project, in Tallahassee, Florida, discovered that primary care was available to poor and uninsured residents from a network of county and federally funded health centers in the city and surrounding rural counties of Florida's Panhandle. But health center patients with complicated or chronic problems had almost no access to specialists or hospital-based treatment. The Reach Out effort, led by James W. Stockwell, a gastroenterologist, bridges that local gap with an extensive network of private specialist physicians willing to donate their services. Through contacts it has cultivated at each referral site, and through computerized case management, the Reach Out project is emerging as an important link between uninsured patients and the resources of the larger medical community.

The project made it possible for Fanny Strickland, a fifty-three-year-old grandmother living alone in a trailer near the Ochlocknee River, to regain the use of her arm and live pain-free for the first time in three years. A benign fatty tumor on her right shoulder had grown to grapefruit size, putting pressure on a joint already damaged by a rotator cuff injury. But Strickland lacked insurance to cover the cost of corrective surgery. By the time the Reach Out project found her, through contacts at public clinics, she had been sleeping upright in a living-room chair for two months, unable to lie down because of the pain. A volunteer orthopedic surgeon with the Reach Out project, Mark E. Fahey, removed the tumor and repaired the torn rotator cuff without pay, and Tallahassee Community Hospital, another Reach Out partner, wrote off the charges.

Stockwell has not found the Reach Out mission to be a hard sell in the Tallahassee area. The project is sponsored by the influential Capital Medical Society, which counts 80 percent of the practicing physicians in greater Tallahassee as members. As for the hospitals, Tallahassee's emergency rooms inevitably wind up with the expensive consequences of medical neglect in the Panhandle—catastrophic strokes that could have been prevented with blood-pressure screening and medication, for example, or similarly preventable diabetic crises. So it has been relatively easy to persuade them of the cost-effectiveness of donating services to patients referred by the Reach Out project. The key, according to Stockwell, is managing the distribution of the uninsured caseload equitably and making assignments on the basis of what each volunteer physician, laboratory, or hospital can reasonably handle. He thinks of the Reach Out project as a neutral organizing mechanism for voluntarism.

As in Tallahassee, most Reach Out grantees have discovered the importance of community partners—hospitals, health departments, civic organizations, social service agencies, and elected and business leaders—in doing the job effectively. Physicians are essential, no question, and not solely for the medical care they provide. They are proving to be a significant asset to the projects politically as well, because of the entrée—and clout—they have with decision makers in their communities. Still, those projects which started out believing that they could solve the problem of health care access simply by harnessing the skills and the good will of doctors quickly revised their thinking.

"Medicine today is a team sport," said B. Dale Magee, an obstetrician, who is the president of the Worcester, Massachusetts, District Medical Society, one of the sponsors of a Reach Out project in that industrial city. "A doctor can do only so much if the patient can't afford to fill the prescription or pay for diagnostic tests or follow through on anything else."

So in both the planning and implementation phases, Reach Out grantees have spent more time than anticipated cataloguing local health resources and potentially relevant community services such as transportation and housing, and even literacy and translation services. In effect, the Reach Out project endeavors to become the thread that binds up holes in the local health care safety net.

Of course, that is what President Clinton hoped to do nationally with the Health Security Act. But if anything certain can be said about American health care in the 1990s, it is that times change. The optimistic environment in which Reach Out was launched in 1993 was history by the time the first twenty-two grantees got their money. Having proposed models that they saw as temporary bridges for the uninsured until some universal payment system was in place, the project leaders suddenly found themselves to be virtually the only ones in their communities still talking about the needs of the underserved. Only two months after the first grants were awarded, in August 1994, Congress threw in the towel on health reform. Bitterly divided party leaders called press conferences to proclaim the death of the entire health reform movement and confer partisan blame for its demise.

Those in the second round of grantees were only slightly better off. They had the benefit of knowing that there would be no quick solution to the problems of underserved patients, but they had no way of anticipating the rapidity with which managed care, mergers, and other market forces would upend the traditional structure and relationships in their health care communities. One Reach Out physician, busy signing up volunteers among her largely fee-for-service colleagues, was stunned by the reaction of these colleagues and, in some cases, personal friends, when her physician group became one of the first in the area to sign a managed care contract. The next time she was doing rounds at the local hospital, she found her name posted on the door of the doctors' lounge under the heading "Wall of Shame." Needless to say, that incident set recruiting back a bit, until the project was able to persuade physicians of the neutrality of its goals.

THREE CASES

Perhaps the best way to understand the ups and downs of Reach Out is by looking at a few projects closely to see how the world has treated them. Asheville, North Carolina; Lincoln, Nebraska; and Sacramento, California, all have Reach Out projects, in distinctly different health care environments. How they've ridden out the storm of the last two years offers lessons in flexibility, shrewd management, and sheer stubbornness of purpose—qualities that in Reach Out are proving to be at least equal in importance to the health reform model being tested.

Asheville, North Carolina: Where Some Market Forces Turn out to Be Friendly

On the surface, Asheville does not seem to lack for anything. A picturesque city tucked into a hollow of the Blue Ridge Mountains, it has been a tourist mecca since the turn of the century. Today, the Blue Ridge Parkway brings thousands of visitors, some to stay in Asheville's Victorian bed-and-breakfasts and poke through its craft shops, others bent on hiking in nearby Great Smoky Mountain National Park.

The city's medical resources are as abundant as the local scenery. Asheville's hospitals are referral centers for much of western North Carolina. Some 460 physicians practice in the city and surrounding Buncombe County. If they were to focus solely on serving their own community, that would be a ratio of one physician for every 413 residents.

Not everyone in Buncombe County benefits from this medical abundance, however. Nine percent of the adults lack health insurance, as do 13 percent of the households with children. Cost and lack of public transportation in the county are the major barriers to timely medical care. Yet uninsured patients are more than twice as likely as those with private health insurance to use hospital emergency rooms, the most costly setting for treatment. Out of a hundred thousand annual emergency room visits, one third were made by uninsured patients, representing a significant loss to the city's hospitals. The hospitals estimated that 25–40 percent of these visits could have been handled more appropriately in a physician's office.

These were among the findings of extensive community surveys conducted by the leaders of Asheville's Reach Out project: Suzanne E. Landis, an internist; Philip C. Davis, an obstetrician-gynecologist; and their sponsor, the Buncombe County Medical Society. They also documented subtler access barriers. Although Asheville has what many would consider a doctor surplus, the vast majority are specialists. Fewer than a hundred are in primary care fields. Their caseload is heavy. Even insured patients report waits of two months or more for appointments. The market in Asheville is still overwhelmingly fee-for-service; managed care accounts for only about 8 percent of insured patients.

So the Reach Out project, called Project Access, had some immediate obstacles to achieving its stated goal of improving medical care for uninsured patients who are below 200 percent of the federal poverty level: a lopsided four-to-one ratio of specialists to primary care physicians, a fairly isolated rural population, and no obvious source of money to cover the ancillary costs of the project. Physician volunteers were the conceptual mainstay of Project Access, but how could it meet needs for medicine, diagnostic tests, and even hospitalization? Community sources of health-related financial support were limited, and what there was had been claimed for years by the major health care institutions in Asheville: the hospitals and the local health department.

But Project Access also had some things going for it. Members of the Buncombe County Medical Society were concerned about access to health care even before President Clinton made it a national issue. Since 1991, about a hundred of them had volunteered regularly at a free three-night-a-week clinic cosponsored by the Asheville Buncombe Community Christian Ministry. And the city's two private hospitals, though competitors, both supported the clinic with some funding as well as free laboratory and x-ray services. Finally, Buncombe County's governing commissioners had long recognized that indigent health care was a community responsibility. Their traditional means of providing such care, however, was to allocate about $600,000 a year to the hospitals to offset losses from charity care and to augment the budget of the Buncombe County Health Department.

One of the first things Project Access helped to change was those funding priorities. Presented with the project's survey results, the county commissioners decided in fiscal 1996 to shift their subsidy from hospital bad debt to programs aimed at preventing serious illness and improving community health. "Six hundred thousand looks like a lot of money, but it doesn't go very far when you give it to hospitals," said Tom Sobol, a county commissioner for twelve years.

The commissioners earmarked $75,000 for prescription drugs for patients certified by Project Access, a sum that will increase to $250,000 by 1998. They also allocated $20,000 to the free clinic. Project Access, meanwhile, recruited more physician volunteers so that hours at the clinic could be expanded. The project also significantly increased the number of doctors willing to see Project Access patients at no cost in their offices. By doubling the number of physicians participating in indigent care—a goal it expects to achieve by 1998—Project Access estimates that seventy-three hundred of the roughly nine thousand uninsured Buncombe County residents with incomes below twice the federal poverty line will have access to regular medical care.

Project Access began its work with a community advisory board of more than one hundred Buncombe County health care and business leaders, as well as consumers. The size of the group was unwieldy, to say the least. At an early planning meeting, in the largest conference room available, it still wasn't possible to get everyone a place at the table, and some had to sit in folding chairs with papers balanced in their laps, or stand along the wall. Predictably, in those first meetings participants clung to the narrow interests of their constituency, the business community desiring to reduce the cost of health benefits, the health department determined to preserve programs. Yet the arduous effort required to achieve consensus paid off. The dimensions of the access problems in Buncombe County and their possible solutions became well understood by community leaders outside the health care establishment. Improving access to health care was thus transformed from the pet project of philanthropically minded doctors to a broad-based community undertaking.

This inclusionary process has also positioned the project to benefit from the latest market convulsion in Asheville. Out of the blue, the city's two private hospitals—Memorial Mission Hospital (418 beds) and St. Joseph's Hospital (292 beds)—announced in late 1995 that they were, in effect, merging. To win an antitrust exemption under North Carolina law, the hospitals had to promise that $74.2 million in projected operational savings over five years would be passed on to needy patients in low-cost or no-cost health services. The hospitals, now known as the Mission + St. Joseph's Health System, can count free care in their emergency rooms as part of that public benefit. But if institutional charity falls short of $74.2 million, the hospitals must contribute the balance to community-based health programs, according to the Certificate of Public Advantage (COPA) issued by the North Carolina attorney general's office.

Landis believes that Project Access presents an ideal vehicle for the hospitals to document compliance. They have already assumed a "much more proactive role" toward the project, she noted, prodded not only by requirements of the COPA but also by the commissioners' surprise reallocation of indigent care dollars. The hospitals have also dropped their case-by-case posture on charity and are now committed to waiving hospital inpatient and outpatient charges for all Project Access patients.

"Many of us are cautiously optimistic, especially with the COPA," Landis said of Project Access. "Anything the hospitals donate—staff, time, services, money—helps them satisfy their COPA requirements. So we become useful to each other." Ultimately, the biggest beneficiaries may be the medically needy residents of Buncombe County.

Lincoln, Nebraska: When the Best-Laid Plans Meet Medicaid Managed Care

Like most good ideas, the Reach Out proposal of the Lancaster County Medical Society was a simple one. Even better, it had been field tested. The model was a successful Medicaid access project under way since 1991 in Lincoln, the county seat. Referral systems, record keeping, patient follow-up—all had been designed and refined. Over three years, nearly nine thousand Medicaid patients had been matched with private physicians, 84 percent of whom signed up with the program. Before that, physician participation in Medicaid had been so low that new Medicaid patients couldn't get an appointment. In effect, their insurance cards were useless outside hospital emergency rooms and a few public clinics.

The Lancaster County effort was a partnership between the medical society, the county health department, and the state social services agency. The core of the program was a telephone hotline, staffed by public health nurses who assessed the immediacy of callers' medical needs and matched patients with doctors. People with transportation problems were given cab vouchers. Paperwork burdens on physicians were minimized, and there were few reimbursement snafus—a chronic complaint about the state's Medicaid program. Doctors also were happy that the load of these relatively low-paying patients was being equitably shared by most of their colleagues.

Buoyed by success, the Lancaster County Medical Society and the county health department decided to expand the program to include physicians, Medicaid patients, and low-income uninsured residents of fifteen rural counties surrounding Lincoln. Their winning application for a Reach Out grant in 1994 described how access problems in those counties were worse than what Lincoln's Medicaid patients ever experienced. Doctors were few and widely scattered, poverty was widespread, and the public health infrastructure was almost nonexistent. At the time, Nebraska ranked dead last among the states in per capita spending for public health. Twelve of the sixteen target counties were either wholly or partly classified as medically underserved areas, and four counties were areas that had a health professional shortage, federally defined by a ratio of more than thirty-five hundred people for every doctor.

The Reach Out project, called Community Access to Coordinated Healthcare, or CATCH, and led by a rural physician, Darroll J. Loschen, planned to tie these counties into the referral service already established in Lancaster County. It would offer overburdened rural practitioners the resources of specialists in Lincoln as well as support from nurses and social workers in the five counties with public health and social service offices. In effect, the project would pull together a regional network of public and private health care providers in order to make medical services more accessible, regardless of where needy patients lived.

The planners overlooked one small but critical detail: the determination of Nebraska's political leaders to be part of the managed care revolution sweeping the country. The state legislature laid the groundwork in 1993, mandating managed care for Medicaid recipients. But it delayed the implementation of this plan for two years, pending the report of a study commission on the best models for Nebraska's diverse regions. The proud architects of Lincoln's Medicaid access project, now Reach Out leaders, were confident that their low-cost, public/private model would win state approval, and they built that assumption into the design of the rural expansion.

In awarding contracts, however, state officials were influenced less by track records than by their own insecurities about whether they knew enough to manage managed care in-house, according to Sen. Don Wesley, chairman of the Nebraska legislature's Health and Human Services Committee. The state social services agency, which had authority over the Medicaid contracts, opted in late 1994 to invite bids from national managed care companies, citing their expertise in other states. One of these commercial bidders won the Medicaid contract in Lincoln, effectively shutting down the medical society/health department referral system.

"As a state, we were really dazzled by the big corporate managed care companies," says Wesley, whose committee created Nebraska's managed care mandate but lost control over its implementation. "We didn't have enough confidence to build upon what we already had."

The decision was a severe blow to the Reach Out project, which, having lost its base in Lincoln, now had to figure out how to improve access with only the meager resources of the rural counties.

"We began talking to the doctors, to county commissioners, the nurses in the health department offices, and anybody else we could get to sit down with us to figure out what could be done," said Natalie Clark, the executive director of the Lancaster County Medical Society and comanager of the Reach Out project. "We were very cognizant that we could not be the people from Lincoln marching in and telling people what to do."

Project leaders discovered that Nebraska's rural physicians, unlike their urban counterparts, were quite isolated from one another, many of them working long hours in solo practices. The doctors also knew very little about managed care. One of the first things the project did was to invite all the rural doctors to an informational meeting on managed care. There, project leaders explained how better coordination with community-based public health and social services could expand their capacity for taking care of Medicaid patients. Uninsured patients—and there were significant numbers among the farm and processing-plant workers in these small towns—could also benefit from these services. The Reach Out project offered to play the coordinating and referral role pioneered in Lincoln, while simultaneously acquainting needy patients with other health services in their communities, such as free immunization clinics and lead screenings. A toll-free phone line, answered by local public health nurses, was established. Meanwhile, the physicians organized the South East Rural Physicians Alliance, to work collectively with the Reach Out project.

An additional purpose was to educate themselves about managed care and political developments in health care at the state and national levels. Having been burned once, the Reach Out participants did not want to lose what they built in rural Nebraska because of a disconnect with decision makers in the capital. Medicaid managed care was implemented in urban areas only in 1995, and the deadline for the rest of the state was set for 1997.

The Nebraska project's Phoenix-like tenacity is being rewarded these days with political leaders' new interest in public-private partnerships. The managed care companies that won Medicaid contracts in 1995 have not had an easy time of it. Patient enrollment was slower than promised, and the companies have been publicly criticized for failing to contract with enough physicians to manage the caseload. Commercial managed care companies also have shown little interest in Nebraska's rural areas, where people working without health insurance on ranches and farms far outnumber those eligible for Medicaid.

"The upshot of all that we have experienced is a realization that the delivery systems of these services have to be community-based— exactly as the original Lincoln project developed," Senator Wesley says. "The big national experts can bring good ideas; I don't want to blame them for our mistakes. But I think we're beginning to realize that we may be smarter about how to implement these ideas in Nebraska."

Sacramento, California: Where the $64,000 Question Is "Who's the Boss?"

Two historic events have given Sacramento a claim to fame beyond the boundaries of California. One was the Gold Rush of 1849, which made the city a destination point for adventurers, cardsharps, dream-ers, and scalawags from around the globe. The other was the managed care revolution of the 1990s, which by mid-decade had bestowed on Sacramento the distinction of being the nation's most highly managed health care market. Some 90 percent of the insured population are enrolled in health maintenance organizations. No other urban area comes close.

The reasons for the popularity of managed care with residents of Sacramento are various, and not entirely a matter of personal choice. Kaiser Permanente established itself in the city in the 1960s and became a major provider of care to state employees, who are numer-ous in the California capital. Three nearby military bases with thou-sands of civilian employees also contracted with HMOs, making these enterprises the largest players in the private health care market. Finally, in 1992 the state legislature authorized the gradual movement of 5,750,000 Medicaid beneficiaries (the $17 billion California program is called Medi-Cal) into managed care. Four experimental imple-mentation models were designed, and Sacramento County was cho-sen as one of the first test sites in 1994. The Medi-Cal contracts, covering 160,000 beneficiaries, wiped out the last major pocket of fee-for-service medicine in Sacramento. It also intensified competition in a market now dominated by five major physician organizations and their affiliated hospital systems.

The result is that individual doctors have very little say in how busi-ness is done or in how they spend their time. As employees or part-ners in medical groups of thirty or more physicians, many of them are not at liberty, say, to take an afternoon off to volunteer at a free clinic, or accept an uninsured patient into their office practice for free treat-ment. And with so many physicians locked into closed systems of care for members only, the uninsured have few options outside the nine public clinics run by the county health agency.

The staff of those nine clinics, however, was severely reduced by budget cuts in 1992. Hours and days of operation were curtailed. Grow-ing numbers of the sick poor were turned away because there weren't enough physicians to see them. One clinic slated for closure was the Capitol Health Center, the only health care provider in Alkali Flats, an impoverished inner city neighborhood of about thirty-three thou-sand people, many of whom are unemployed, disabled, or homeless.

As medical director of the county clinics, Glennah Trochet was acutely aware of the crisis. A family practitioner, she also was a member of the local Sacramento-El Dorado Medical Society. The dual role led to her 1994 Reach Out proposal to increase the capacity of the public clinics by augmenting the staff with volunteer private physicians. The medical society sponsored the project, called SPIRIT (Sacramento Physicians Initiative to Reach Out, Innovate, and Teach), and the three major hospital systems were recruited as collaborators.

In a fee-for-service market, the support of these key health care institutions would have provided entrée to medical staffs as well as the possibility of funding and donated supplies and services. But in Sacramento, physicians admitting patients to the hospitals owe their first allegiance to their medical group. Even those with control over their schedules may be so pressed by managed care production goals that the choice to volunteer has significant consequences for income. Sacramento also has a surplus of specialists, while its primary care physicians are swamped by the gatekeeper responsibilities that managed care confers on them.

On top of this is the cutthroat nature of the competition in Sacramento. SPIRIT board meetings are one of the few places where representatives of the hospital systems and physician groups sit together in anything that resembles common purpose. The project has the delicate task of trying to create a communitywide network in the name of service to a population that represents no market advantage to any of the competing participants. It was an uneasy alliance at first, and there continues to be tension about whether one group is donating more than the other.

"There is a cost to voluntarism," one high-ranking administrator pointed out. "To the extent that you contribute more than your competitor, you weaken your position." Another said, "Even if we personally believe in this mission, which frankly is the glue that holds SPIRIT together, all of us have to report to bean counters in our own organizations, some of whom aren't even based in Sacramento."

In short, SPIRIT has to sell the message of altruism in an environment where the incomes of prospective physician volunteers are plummeting, and even the institutions cannot anticipate what new belt-tightening will be called for a few months hence. For SPIRIT, the consequences of such market instability are direct and profound. Early in the planning year, the project lost an enthusiastic and highly placed backer in one hospital system when that system eliminated her entire department as part of a cost-cutting reorganization. Two members of

SPIRIT's original governing board were gone inside of a year because their jobs were eliminated.

Yet there are traditions of community service in Sacramento's health care establishment that lie beneath the surface of the current market turbulence. Some physicians have found ways within their complex organizations to carve out time for volunteering. The Capitol Health Center in Alkali Flats now has seven volunteers. It also was saved from closing in 1993 by cash contributions from two of the hospital systems.

Trochet says the setbacks of the first year have made SPIRIT leaders more sophisticated about tailoring traditional volunteer recruitment methods to the managed care environment. The project still appeals to individual physicians, but it is also targeting medical group managers, challenging them to come up with structural innovations that encourage voluntarism. Release time without financial penalty is one concept, in organizations where physicians are employees. And the message is conveyed in new language. Thom Atkins, a SPIRIT board member and chief operating officer of a one-hundred-member multispecialty group, bases his pitch to members on the cost/volume idea of managed care. "My approach is not to go to just the good people I know and ask them to do this," he said. "My approach has been to say to the group, 'Hey, if every one of you donated four hours every six months we could staff one of these clinics entirely on our own.'"

Finally, a new development in California's fast-paced health care revolution may add some fiscal glue to the SPIRIT alliance. A state law that took effect in 1995 requires nonprofit health care institutions to quantify community contributions justifying their tax-exempt status. As in Asheville, North Carolina, the Sacramento Reach Out project is positioned to help local hospitals comply with that requirement by documenting the monetary value of whatever the hospitals contribute to SPIRIT to help improve access for medically needy residents.

CONCLUSION

As The Robert Wood Johnson Foundation prepared to launch Reach Out, a nagging uncertainty dogged the planners. Would anyone apply for a grant?

Private physicians—the group from which Reach Out leaders were expected to emerge—were not a happy bunch in 1993. They had been handled roughly by the polemicists of national health reform, denounced for excessive fees and lavish lifestyles while thirty-seven million uninsured Americans went without care. The rhetorical bashing came as many doctors were beginning to experience a reality that belied their public portrayal: declining incomes and increasing workloads brought on by managed care. There were, of course, doctors who fit the public stereotype. But the greater number—like the ethical, hard-working core of any profession—did not. Many of them had consistently, albeit quietly, upheld medicine's altruistic traditions, volunteering in clinics, writing off bills, and using their influence in hospitals and elsewhere to see that poor patients were cared for.

Still, more than one observer predicted the initiative would be dead on arrival, a nice idea shelved for lack of interest. But the opposite occurred. An unexpectedly large number of applicants responded to the Foundation's published request for proposals. That response, and the more than two thousand colleagues these physician leaders have recruited to the effort, form the primary lesson of Reach Out so far: voluntarism, even in these bottom-line-driven times, is still a powerful force within the health care professions.

The imperatives of the bottom line, however, cannot be ignored if Reach Out projects are to achieve significance beyond their philanthropic origins. This is the harder road ahead for Reach Out. On the most basic level, project leaders have discovered that appeals to busy colleagues, hospitals, and other providers to "do the right thing" don't go very far without an organizational structure to effectively channel contributions. Even the most good-hearted individuals and corporate and government partners are going to do a hard-headed analysis of the risks and benefits of participation. Reach Out leaders must be prepared to make their case in those terms. In Asheville, this has meant poring through complex legal documents of a hospital merger in order to find a sustaining niche for Reach Out. In Sacramento, it has meant analyzing the rapidly changing structure of health care decision making. In Lincoln, it has meant learning how to talk politics with the pros at the State Capitol. Reach Out's physician leaders frequently refer to how much they have had to learn—painfully, sometimes—about the workings of the health care system. Beyond the patients Reach Out projects serve, these lessons hold promise for illuminating the process of reform.

CHAPTER TWO

~ Improving the Health Care Workforce

Perspectives from Twenty-Four Years' Experience

Stephen L. Isaacs
Lewis G. Sandy
Steven A. Schroeder

Editors' Introduction

Today's health care workforce, about eleven million strong, includes people working in jobs ranging from laboratory technician to nurse and from speech pathologist to physician. It is the fastest growing segment of the nation's labor market, employing one out of every ten workers.

Typically, the Foundation looks at its programs one at a time. This chapter is a rare instance of stepping back and looking at the entire body of the Foundation's efforts in one specific area. This overview provides a broad-based perspective of a strategy that has lasted nearly twenty-five years, and it offers insights about the value of the strategy.

The chapter represents the effort of two senior Foundation officials and one outside analyst to make sense of what the Foundation has done and to examine the strengths and weaknesses of a large, long-term investment strategy. The lead author, Stephen L. Isaacs, is president

---

This chapter expands upon ideas initially published by the authors in *Health Affairs*, Summer 1996, pp. 279–295.

of the Center for Health and Social Policy in Pelham, New York. Both Steven A. Schroeder, president of the Foundation, and Lewis G. Sandy, executive vice president of the Foundation, have had a long interest in, and have written about, workforce issues.

As the chapter notes, the impact of the Foundation's workforce programs is difficult to evaluate. Neither individually nor in the aggregate do they represent a large share of the programs, and other forces, that shape the health care workforce. Such programs often attempt to shape a system by supporting individuals, and it is hard to disentangle the many factors that produce effective professionals, let alone an entire workforce. Despite these analytical difficulties, the authors do come to some reasoned conclusions. More important, we hope that the chapter stimulates thinking about new possibilities and new challenges in this important area.

T he Robert Wood Johnson Foundation began operating as a national philanthropy in 1972. It was the year that Henry Kissinger and Le Duc Tho held secret peace negotiations in Paris, Richard Nixon was elected to a second term, and many people thought that national health insurance was right around the corner. Surveys conducted in the early 1970s indicated that access to basic ambulatory care was the nation's number one health care concern. Such concern attracted the immediate attention of the new foundation, and in its 1972 annual report David Rogers, the Foundation's first president, noted the relationship between access to services and the health care workforce:

> The uneven availability of continuing medical care of acceptable quality is one of the most serious problems we face today. The problem is twofold. First, there are too few health resources in rural and urban poverty areas. Thus, we have too many people—particularly our poor, our elderly, and our isolated—lacking ready access to appropriate services. Second, the specialty balance of physicians and their associated personnel is significantly out of line with needs. There is a sharp shortage of those who deliver primary care and increasing evidence to suggest a relative oversupply of physicians in certain medical and surgical specialties.[1]

To increase Americans' access to a physician or some other health care professional, and to prepare for national health insurance, the Foundation made a commitment to expanding and improving the health care workforce—a commitment that continues to this day. The Foundation has funded programs to increase the number of health professionals who can provide primary care to communities in need: generalist physicians, nurse practitioners, physician assistants, and family dentists. In addition, it launched fellowship programs to develop a cadre of health care professionals with interdisciplinary knowledge and breadth of vision who could be leaders in shaping health care policy. Since 1972, the Foundation has allocated $520 million—more than one out of every five dollars it has awarded—to workforce programs. National programs carried out at a number of sites have received $419 million; these are listed and described in

Exhibit 2.1 at the end of this chapter. Another $101 million has been given in ad hoc, or single site, grants.

The Foundation does not, of course, act in isolation. Other foundations also fund programs to make the health care workforce more responsive to national needs. For example, the W. K. Kellogg Foundation was an early supporter of family practice; the Commonwealth Fund supported innovative projects like the WAMI program, designed to bring primary care to underserved communities in Washington, Alaska, Montana, and Idaho; the Kaiser Family Foundation supported faculty fellowships in general internal medicine; and the Pew Charitable Trusts offer health policy fellowships and operate a Health Professions Commission that examines workforce issues.

Governments have also become more active in reshaping the workforce. Many states now promote primary care initiatives within their own borders. The federal government, through Titles VII and VIII of the Public Health Service Act, supports the education of health professionals. Through the National Health Service Corps, it places physicians in underserved areas in return for scholarships or forgiveness of student loans. The federal government currently spends more than $400 million a year in forty-four workforce initiatives that encourage health professionals to study primary care and to practice in underserved areas.[2] Even greater federal funding goes toward specialization and high technology. This includes $6 billion a year that Medicare spends annually for graduate medical education, and $8.5 billion that the National Institutes of Health spend annually for medical research and training.[3]

Then there are market forces—perhaps the most crucial factor in determining what and where health professionals practice. The rise of managed care, for example, is persuading an increasing number of medical students to consider careers as generalists. However, since there are few financial incentives to serve chronically ill, poor, or geographically isolated individuals, managed care may do little to increase access for underserved populations.

Although the resources of any one foundation may be relatively modest in terms of the total available for health care issues, philanthropy can play a unique and catalytic role. Rogers said of this role, "A foundation can offer people, institutions, and communities the opportunity to test a new approach and then give others the chance to prod it, examine it, and see if it fits their particular set of circumstances, and whether it can have yet broader application. Fear of the new is sometimes allayed by taking an idea out of the abstract and seeing it in operation."[4]

1970s WORKFORCE PROGRAMS

Primary Care Physicians

Since its earliest days, the Foundation has given high priority to promoting primary care and making it a more attractive career for physicians. In the 1970s, it launched programs (Figure 2.1) intended to attract top internists and pediatricians to primary care, so as to enhance the credibility and the standing of primary care in the medical community. This approach—training a small number of key individuals, particularly academics, to serve as agents of change in a high-priority area—was to serve as a model for the Foundation. The *Primary Care Residency Program,* begun in 1973, gave training in primary care to general pediatric residents and internal medicine residents at nine hospitals and outpatient clinics. Six years later, the Foundation began the *General Pediatric Academic Development Program,* which awarded two-year fellowships to prepare pediatric faculty members to conduct research on the more common childhood illnesses such as ear infections that were not, at the time, covered in medical school curricula. The third program, the *Family Practice Fellowship Program,* attempted to establish a firmer academic base for family medicine by training a small core of highly respected faculty members. Begun in 1978, it complemented the federal government's short-term fellowships in family practice by offering two-year postresidency fellowships in family medicine.

These three programs helped develop the field of primary care, giving it more respectability in academic medicine. The Primary Care Residency Program served as a model for the federal government, which began funding primary care training for internists and pediatricians in 1977. The General Pediatric Academic Development Program led to the inclusion of general pediatrics as a normal part of pediatricians' training. An evaluation of the Family Practice Fellowship Program found that four years after it ended 65 percent of the graduates held medical school appointments and more than 90 percent, including those not affiliated with a medical school, spent some of their time teaching.

Figure 2.1.   Foundation National Workforce Programs Begun
              in the 1970s.

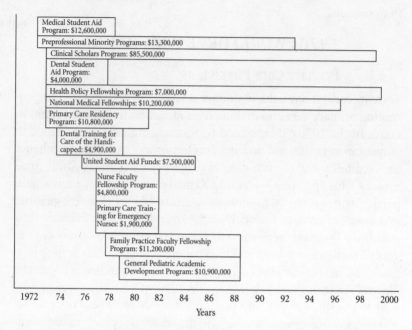

Medical Student Aid Program: $12,600,000
Preprofessional Minority Programs: $13,300,000
Clinical Scholars Program: $85,500,000
Dental Student Aid Program: $4,000,000
Health Policy Fellowships Program: $7,000,000
National Medical Fellowships: $10,200,000
Primary Care Residency Program: $10,800,000
Dental Training for Care of the Handicapped: $4,900,000
United Student Aid Funds: $7,500,000
Nurse Faculty Fellowship Program: $4,800,000
Primary Care Training for Emergency Nurses: $1,900,000
Family Practice Faculty Fellowship Program: $11,200,000
General Pediatric Academic Development Program: $10,900,000

1972   74   76   78   80   82   84   86   88   90   92   94   96   98   2000

Years

Nurse Practitioners, Physician Assistants, and Health Associates

When the Foundation began its philanthropic efforts, it recognized that if health care were to be made accessible to underserved populations, health professionals other than physicians would have to be trained to deliver primary care. As a result, it began supporting the training of nurse practitioners and physician assistants in the early 1970s, a time when both fields were in their infancy. Initially, grants were made to a number of demonstration programs. The Utah Valley Hospital in Provo, for example, received funds to establish a network of rural clinics that would be staffed by nurse practitioners backed up by physicians who flew in every week. At the same time, the Foundation supported several pilot programs to train physician assistants.

Acceptance of nurse practitioners did not come easily. (Physician assistants were less threatening to people, since their profession grew out of efforts within the medical profession, and they worked directly under the supervision of doctors.) Many people in the medical community saw nurse practitioners as unqualified upstarts eager to encroach on the territory of physicians. To placate these concerns and give credibility to advanced-degree primary care nursing, the Foundation adopted two approaches to bring nurse-practitioner training into the mainstream of graduate nursing education. In the mid–1970s, it awarded ad hoc grants to six nursing schools to establish primary care training for nurse practitioners at the master's degree level. Next, it initiated a *Nurse Faculty Fellowship Program* to develop a core of nursing educators who would be able to train nurse practitioners at the master's level. Between 1977 and 1982, ninety-nine fellows—the pioneers in a movement that led to the acceptance of nurse-practitioner training as an integral part of graduate nursing education—completed the program.

Before the Foundation established its successful nursing programs, it provided funds to The Johns Hopkins University in 1973 to establish a school of health services that would train a new class of health professional—similar in some ways to physician assistants—called health associates. These newly minted professionals were to be the model for the delivery of primary care services at a time when the debut of national health insurance seemed imminent. However, the school closed after only four classes had graduated.

This was the Foundation's most visible workforce failure: an admittedly high-risk idea that, if successful, might have had a major impact on the delivery of health services. In retrospect, it may have been unrealistic to expect a medical school whose reputation depended on training specialists to throw its support behind an approach to health care that would rely on people who were not physicians. Moreover, the timing for such a program was simply not right. National health insurance was not enacted in the 1970s, and the huge infusions of federal money to train physician assistants and other health professionals as part of health care reform never materialized. Within the university, the new school had little political leverage. Given these factors, it is not surprising that when the university suffered a budget crisis in the seventies and the Foundation's funding also ended, Johns Hopkins decided not to commit any more of its scarce resources to the school.

With this exception, the Foundation's early nurse practitioner and physician assistant programs have been among its more successful undertakings. Its funding helped establish these two fields as viable career options at a time when the idea of such programs was under attack. The Foundation decided to withdraw its support for these programs in the late 1970s, after Congress began earmarking money to train nurse practitioners, physician assistants, and generalist physicians. The Foundation reasoned that once the models it had helped develop were adopted by the federal government, it should move on to new endeavors. Although nurse practitioners and physician assistants still faced formidable legal, political, and financial obstacles, for twelve years beginning in 1982 the Foundation did not develop any new national programs directed toward these health professionals.

Dentistry

Another field that attracted the early attention of the Foundation was dentistry. The *Program for Training Dentists in the Care of Handicapped Patients,* 1974–1979, led to the inclusion of dentistry for handicapped patients in the standard dental school curriculum. The *Dental Research Scholars Program* aimed at developing a cadre of dental faculty members knowledgeable in health care services and administration. It awarded two-year postdoctoral fellowships for research in dental health services. The Foundation did not fund any new national workforce programs for dentists after 1982, although it did provide partial support for an Institute of Medicine study on the future of dental education and continued to provide ad hoc grants to the dental profession.

Fellowships

The Foundation also has sought to improve the American health care climate by developing health professionals—primarily physicians—who understand health services, the social sciences, and health policy making, and who could become leaders in their home institutions, professional societies, and state and federal government. To train these leaders, the Foundation established two fellowship programs.

Established by the Commonwealth Fund and the Carnegie Corporation in 1969, the *Clinical Scholars Program* was taken over and expanded by The Robert Wood Johnson Foundation shortly after the Foundation became a national philanthropy. This program, which continues to flourish, gives young physicians who are committed to clinical careers the opportunity to acquire skills and knowledge in areas such as epidemiology, economics, law, biostatistics, management, ethics, and anthropology. Currently, thirty-four scholars (eight of whom are funded by the Department of Veterans Affairs) are chosen annually to spend two years studying and conducting research at one of seven leading academic medical centers. Outside evaluators have praised the program as "a national treasure"[5] and "exceptionally influential."[6] Many of its more than seven hundred graduates have become leaders in academic institutions, managed health care programs, and government agencies.

The second program, begun in 1973 and still in operation, is the *Health Policy Fellowships Program.* Every year, it gives six outstanding midcareer health professionals an in-depth look at the federal health policy process. The fellowships begin with a three-month orientation in Washington, D.C., followed by a nine-month placement in the office of a senator, representative, or senior member of an executive department.

1980s WORKFORCE PROGRAMS

In the 1980s, the federal government turned away from the role it had played since the 1930s in addressing the nation's social problems. Rising health care costs became a national concern; the maldistribution of the health care workforce worsened, particularly as more young physicians chose careers in medical specialties. During this period, the Foundation solidified its commitment to training minority health professionals, developed national programs to strengthen the nursing profession, and established a new fellowship program for health care finance (Figure 2.2).

Minority Physicians

The Foundation has allocated more than $100 million to date to minority health professionals. Although this commitment began with its very first program—medical school scholarships for women, students from rural areas, and minorities—it was in the mid-1980s that the Foundation launched its first national initiatives to bring more minorities into the health professions. What the Foundation hopes to achieve is increased access: if everyone is to have access to medical care, there must be more minority health professionals, for studies show that they choose careers in primary care, serve other minorities, and provide care to poor patients to a greater degree than nonminority

Figure 2.2.   Foundation National Workforce Programs Begun in the 1980s.

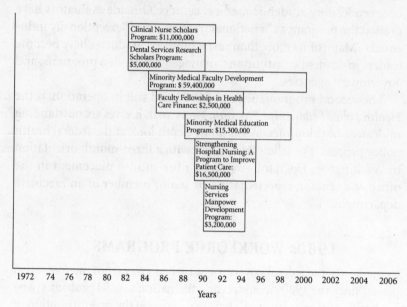

1972	74	76	78	80	82	84	86	88	90	92	94	96	98	2000	2002	2004	2006

Years

physicians. African Americans, Mexican Americans, Native Americans, and mainland Puerto Ricans make up 22 percent of the United States population, but only a small proportion of the health care workforce.

In addition to its early scholarship programs for needy minority medical students, the Foundation addressed the fact that many minority applicants had not been adequately prepared to enter medical school. Many of these students had not taken the right premed courses and had not been adequately prepared for the Medical College Admission Test (MCAT); as a result, they could not compete successfully for admission with other college students. To overcome these disadvantages, the Foundation supported a wide variety of enrichment programs for minority college students in the 1970s and early 1980s.

In 1985, a report issued by the Educational Testing Service found that summer programs increased the chances that minority students would be accepted into medical school. The Foundation combined its various enrichment programs into one national program, the *Minority Medical Education Program,* which continues today. Guided by a mentor, students learn about medical care and research, take courses in math and science, and are counseled in practical matters such as how to complete a medical school application and improve their interview skills. Currently, eight academic medical centers participate, each providing a six-week summer program for approximately 125 minority college students. An in-house evaluation found that the summer enrichment program doubles a student's chances of being admitted to a medical school.[7]

Even highly qualified and well-prepared minority students have been hesitant to apply to medical schools that did not have minority faculty members who could ease the difficulties that minority students sometimes encounter. So the *Minority Medical Faculty Development Program* was developed to increase the number of full-time minority faculty members in nonminority medical schools. Begun in 1984, this program helps promising junior faculty members who are committed to academic careers move up the academic ladder by offering them four-year postdoctoral research fellowships. Research can be in the biomedical, clinical, or health services area. Initially, eight fellows a year were appointed; this number was increased to twelve in 1991. A recent evaluation concluded that the program played a pivotal role in developing the potential for advancement of its program graduates who have remained in academic medicine.[8]

The Foundation also supported faculty development at the nation's traditionally black medical colleges. The bulk of Foundation support has gone to Meharry Medical College in Nashville, Tennessee, primarily to strengthen its faculty.

Nursing

During the 1980s, the Foundation launched a number of programs to improve the training of nurses and to alleviate a critical nursing shortage. The first of these was the *Clinical Nurse Scholars Program,* which addressed a serious problem of hospital nursing: college-trained nurses did not have the practical experience needed to provide adequate patient care. The Foundation designed a program, patterned on the Clinical Scholars Program, to prepare a cadre of nursing school faculty for careers combining clinical practice, research, and management.

These clinical nurse scholars would provide a base of notable and credible faculty members who would be capable of bridging the gap between nursing education, with its focus on research, and nursing practice, with its focus on patient care and management.

As the program was originally designed, nine midcareer fellows were to be chosen every year to conduct clinical or health sciences research. The first nurse scholars were selected in 1982. As it developed, however, the program shifted direction and became a basic research fellowship program for postdoctoral students. This led the Foundation to reconsider the program, and to end it three years earlier than planned. The last group of fellows completed its studies in 1991.

The 1980s witnessed a severe shortage of nurses; a commission established by the Secretary of Health and Human Services characterized this shortage as "real, widespread, and of significant magnitude."[9] In response, the Foundation funded three new national programs. The first, *Strengthening Hospital Nursing: A Program to Improve Patient Care*, was a six-year, $26.8 million effort begun in 1989. Funded jointly with the Pew Charitable Trusts, the program attempted to make hospital nursing a more attractive career choice by restructuring medical and support services around the nursing staff. More than a thousand hospitals and consortiums submitted applications, eighty of which received planning grants, and twenty of which were awarded five-year implementation grants.

The two other programs—the *Nursing Services Manpower Development Program*, begun in 1989, and *Ladders in Nursing Careers*, begun in 1993—aimed at increasing the number of nurses by attracting and supporting disadvantaged students and health care workers who wanted to pursue nursing careers. The seven Nursing Services Manpower Program grantees adopted approaches ranging from counseling minority seventh graders to setting up a cooperative recruitment program among nursing schools to attract minority students. Under the Ladders in Nursing Careers Program, grants were awarded to nine hospital associations to help employees, especially nurses' aides, overcome financial, educational, and other barriers to becoming nurses.

For a variety of reasons, the Foundation has not succeeded in developing a coherent and consistent approach to its nursing programs. Some of the reasons have to do with the characteristics of nursing: the gulf between the academic focus of nursing education and the clinical focus of its practice; three distinct entry levels (diploma, associate degree, and baccalaureate degree) leading to what many employers consider the same job; the lack of agreement about nurses' roles and the skills nurses need to fill their roles; and the recurring scarcity and surplus of nurses.[10]

Other reasons have their roots in the Foundation's approach. Perhaps reflecting the bias of an organization whose three presidents have been internists from academic medical institutions, the Foundation single-mindedly pursued its goal of training primary care physicians. In contrast, its nursing programs addressed short-term labor crises rather than long-term needs; supported activities with diffuse, conflicting, or unclear objectives; and lacked follow-through. The Clinical Nurse Scholars Program was probably terminated prematurely; although it had veered from its original objectives, it might have been redesigned to overcome its problems.[11] The Strengthening Hospital Nursing program had unclear and perhaps unrealistic objectives. Not only did it focus exclusively on process but its twin goals—one having to do with reorganizing hospital care around nursing, the other having to do with improving patient care—were not necessarily compatible. (In addition, it had the misfortune to begin just as many hospitals were laying off nurses in a wave of downsizing.) Similarly, the objectives of the Nursing Services Manpower Training and Ladders in Nursing Careers programs were overly broad: on the one hand they were supposed to increase the supply of nurses, and on the other they were supposed to attract minorities to nursing careers.

Health Care Finance

As health care evolved in the 1980s from the fee-for-service care offered by nonprofit institutions to managed care provided by for-profit entities, and as cost became a public policy issue, it became increasingly clear that health care finance was the key to understanding the system—and perhaps to reforming it. It became equally clear that the number of people who could claim expertise in this complex field was limited. In 1985, the Foundation began its *Program for Faculty Fellowships in Health Care Finance*. It offered thirty-month fellowships to six faculty members a year. An evaluation found that even though the program changed the lives of many of its fellows, its target audience was unclear; for example, it was not clear whether the purpose was to increase the knowledge of professors of health care finance, introduce health policy faculty to financing issues, or train professors of finance in health policy issues. Concern was also raised about the narrowness of an approach that trained faculty in health care financing apart from overall health policy. The program ended in 1994.

1990s WORKFORCE PROGRAMS

The early 1990s were characterized by concern about escalating health care costs, President Clinton's failed attempt to reform the system, and the growth of for-profit managed care. Within the Foundation, a new board chairman took office in 1989, a new president in 1990. These appointments led to a refocusing of the Foundation's workforce programs: renewed emphasis on educating primary care physicians, reinvigorated efforts to train other health care professionals, and concentration on entire systems of health care rather than individual components. At the same time, the Foundation reasserted its commitment to minorities and opened its fellowship programs to a wider group of recipients (Figure 2.3).

Figure 2.3.   Foundation National Workforce Programs Begun in the 1990s.

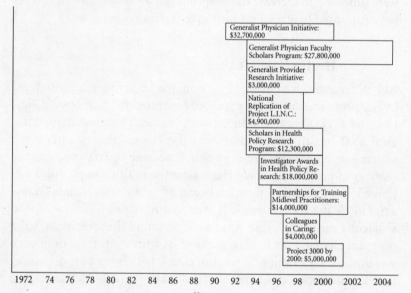

Generalist Physicians

In the early 1990s, as part of a $100 million strategy to improve access to basic health care, the Foundation launched a second cluster of programs to bring primary care into the mainstream of academic medicine and to attract more medical students to general medicine. The goal was no less than to change the thrust and the focus of medical education. Unlike the programs of the 1970s, which added more generalists to the pool of physicians without reducing the number of specialists, these programs sought more fundamental change: shifting the balance between generalists and specialists.

Under the *Generalist Physician Initiative,* the Foundation gave grants to medical schools that made a commitment to training generalist physicians and to increasing the proportion of generalists to specialists they graduated. Working in collaboration with state agencies, HMOs, and other partners, the grantees devised strategies aimed at four critical points in medical education: admissions, undergraduate medical curriculum, residency, and entry into practice. Beginning in 1991, the Foundation awarded planning grants to eighteen medical schools and consortiums, followed by six-year awards to fourteen of them to carry out the programs they had designed. The initiative stimulated a number of innovative partnerships and served as a model for New York and Pennsylvania to develop their own grant programs to increase the supply of primary care physicians.

A parallel program, the *Generalist Physician Faculty Scholars Program,* started in 1993, aimed at increasing the prestige and credibility of generalist faculty members at medical schools. Recognizing that published research is the key to respect and seniority in academia, the program awarded four-year research grants to up to fifteen junior faculty members annually.

In lieu of evaluating each of its programs to encourage generalist medicine, and to place its efforts in a larger context, the Foundation funded the *Generalist Provider Research Initiative,* a five-year program also begun in 1993. Awards were made to carry out research on issues such as how to increase the number of physicians entering the three generalist fields, reduce the number of specialists, and attract more physicians to underserved areas.

Until the managed care revolution changed the way that professionals viewed health care, American medical students looked askance at careers in general medicine. The percentage of medical students selecting one of the three generalist fields—general internal medicine, general pediatrics, and family practice—as their first choice dropped from 36 percent in 1982 to less than 17 percent in 1991 and 1992. But the need for primary care physicians by managed care organizations appears to have reversed that trend. In 1993, the percentage of medical students making one of the general medicine fields their first choice rose to 19 percent; it has continued to rise, reaching 35 percent in 1996.

The extent to which The Robert Wood Johnson Foundation programs contributed to the changed environment is hard to determine. While market forces no doubt played a dominant role, they were augmented and reinforced by the Foundation's efforts. At the least, through its programs and a phenomenon known as the brochure effect,* the Foundation's long commitment helped validate the idea of training generalists, made medical school faculty and administrators more receptive to primary care, and prepared medical schools to teach general medicine.

Physician Assistants, Nurse Practitioners, and Certified Nurse Midwives

Beyond its work with medical schools in training primary care physicians, the Foundation took steps to educate other health professionals who might practice in underserved areas. Unlike the programs of the 1970s, these initiatives involved health care systems: state agencies, HMOs, community organizations, professional schools, and the like. *The Partnerships for Training Program,* started in 1996, required institutions in a region—universities, HMOs, state agencies, employers—to collaborate in the use of nontraditional techniques such as distance learning to train nurse practitioners, certified nurse midwives, and physician assistants in their home communities. Since these health professionals are being educated in the underserved communities where they live, they are expected to practice in those communities when their training is completed.

---

* The brochure effect is a well-recognized phenomenon that is difficult to quantify, by which the announcement of a national program calls attention to a priority area of the Foundation, and institutions that are not currently receiving grants then move in the direction of the national program.

Minority Health Professionals

The 1990s also saw an expansion of the training of minority health care professionals. In part because of the Foundation's Minority Medical Education Program, academically qualified minority students had a good chance of being admitted to medical school. But the number of minority students is small relative to their proportion in the population. To reach a far wider pool at an earlier point in their lives, the Association of American Medical Colleges (AAMC) began *Project 3000 by 2000* in 1991. This program tries to attract and prepare high school students for medical careers. The goal of the AAMC is to more than double—from thirteen hundred to three thousand—the number of underrepresented minority students entering medical school by the year 2000.

In 1994, with Foundation support, the project expanded to include other health professionals. Working in partnerships with colleges, school systems, and communities, ten academic centers offer enrichment courses, collaborate in creating magnet health sciences programs in high schools, provide mentors, and strengthen the science skills of elementary and secondary teachers. As mentioned earlier, the Foundation also is attempting to increase the number of minority nurses through two other programs: the Nursing Services Manpower and the Ladders in Nursing Careers programs.

Expanding Fellowship Opportunities in Health Policy

Responding to changes in the health care system, in the 1990s the Foundation expanded the eligibility requirements for people who might become fellows. At mid-decade, amid concerns that bright junior members of social science faculties were not drawn to health policy research and that senior investigators were not receiving sufficient support, the Foundation initiated two new fellowship programs. Under the *Scholars in Health Policy Research Program,* which started in 1993, twelve two-year postdoctoral fellowships are awarded annually to promising young economists, political scientists, and sociologists. The *Investigator Awards in Health Policy Research,* which began in 1994, broadens the pool of health policy researchers even further: applicants may come from any discipline. The program provides salary support for ten outstanding young researchers or eminent senior scholars for up to three years.

PERSPECTIVES FROM TWENTY-FOUR YEARS OF EXPERIENCE

From its very earliest days, the Foundation had a vision of a health care system that would be available to all Americans. As a result, it funded a multitude of programs to improve the health care workforce in the belief that this would result in more available care. Some, such as the Clinical Scholars Program, succeeded spectacularly. Others, such as the bold attempt to establish a new class of health associates at Johns Hopkins, failed utterly.

Where the Foundation worked with academic medicine, it has been successful. Through its programs with academic medical centers, it has been a major force in developing the field of general internal medicine, in introducing primary care into the medical school curriculum and residency training, and in making medical education more relevant. Perhaps more important than the specific programs it funded, the Foundation served as what one commentator called "a moral compass."[12] It pursued its vision of primary care as the key to health services, even when the idea seemed hopelessly unfashionable.

The Foundation showed similar determination in fostering a core of physicians to assume positions of leadership in the health care field. The Clinical Scholars Program, now nearly a quarter of a century old, is considered to be its flagship program, boasting a large constituency within the Foundation, among the program directors at the schools that train the fellows, and in academic medicine generally. The Foundation has also stayed the course in preparing minority students for medical school and training minority medical faculty.

When it came to nonphysician health professionals, however, the Foundation showed little of the same clear vision and steely devotion that characterized its programs for improving the physician workforce. After taking the lead in developing nurse practitioners and physician assistants as viable professions, it pulled back support in the early 1980s. Its nursing programs have lacked coherence and long-term perspective. The flow of money speaks loudly here: national programs to train physicians consumed 70 percent of the Foundation's workforce budget, leaving 30 percent for training all other health professionals (Figure 2.4).

**Figure 2.4. National Workforce Programs for Physicians
and Other Health Professionals by Dollar Amount and Percentage.**

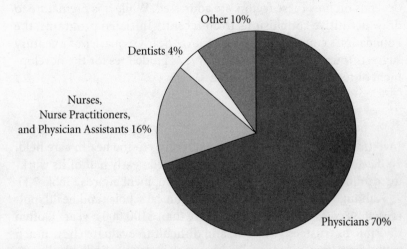

Perhaps reflecting its comfort with academic medical institutions, the Foundation was slow to recognize that the shift in health care from the medical community to corporations and business concerns presented an opportunity to offer training to individuals from disciplines such as economics, management, and law that are not normally associated with health care.

As the twenty-first century approaches, the question is how the nation's workforce programs will respond to a health care system that was barely envisioned in the relatively recent past. Twenty-some years ago, "health maintenance organization" was a concept known to only a smattering of academicians, policy wonks, and health professionals. Now most people with medical needs enter the world of managed care, where large conglomerates buy and sell health services, generalist physicians serve as gatekeepers, and the bottom line is paramount. Government can no longer be counted on to ensure that services are provided for the neediest citizens, and federal subsidies for graduate medical education are threatened. With the graying of the population, more chronic care is provided in homes and outpatient facilities. At the same time, the amount of acute care in hospitals is declining as these services are delivered on an outpatient basis. Advances in communications technology are changing the way information is transmitted and received.

This is the context in which workforce programs intended for the early twenty-first century operate. The *content* of the programs depends on how these factors are addressed. While it is premature to draw definitive conclusions from recently initiated programs, the Foundation's cumulative experience over nearly a quarter of a century suggests four principles that can serve as guidelines for the development of future workforce programs.

Invest in Individuals

Investments in people provide great returns to the health care field. To date, the Foundation has already devoted nearly half of its workforce funds to fellowships and faculty development awards (Table 2.1).

Although these are expensive (each clinical scholar and health policy fellow costs the Foundation more than $100,000 a year[13]), often invisible to trustees and staff, and difficult to evaluate (how much credit, for example, does a fellowship contribute to an individual's success later in life?), they are a productive investment. They give talented individuals the freedom to take risks and enter careers that the market is not yet willing to support.

What's more, there is a professional advantage in being awarded an esteemed fellowship. Such a plum often leads to enhanced career opportunities and to greater influence on the institutions where fellows work, the professional societies to which they belong, and health policy in general. It may be that the Foundation has had more effect on academic medicine and the public policy process indirectly through its fellows and scholars than directly through its institutional support.

Broaden Fellowships to Other Disciplines

As professionals other than physicians play a greater role in health care, fellowship programs should be broadened to include people from a wide range of disciplines. The Foundation's fellowship programs during the 1970s and 1980s reflected the dominance of physicians in the health care system. During these years, the Foundation invested heavily in training physicians, particularly internists. It made a smaller but still substantial investment in nursing and dental fellows.[14] Of the programs initiated in those decades, only the health policy fellowships (which, in practice, have been awarded mainly to physicians) and the faculty fellowships in health care finance were open to a broader range of disciplines.

In the 1990s, the role of business executives, economists, lawyers, and other nonphysicians in shaping health policy has expanded, while the dominance of physicians has diminished. Whatever one might think of this trend, it does offer an opportunity to broaden the network of people who receive fellowships, and indeed, recent Foundation programs have opened up fellowships to individuals from nonmedical, nonnursing disciplines. In light of this change, and in recognition of the changes in the health care sector, it is time to explore an increased focus on training professionals who can play important roles but do not come from disciplines traditionally associated with health care.

Attend to Total Systems

With the rapid and dramatic changes in health services, workforce programs should involve total systems of health care rather than focusing on specific components such as medical centers. In the 1970s, the power to affect health care lay substantially with academic medicine. This led The Robert Wood Johnson Foundation to concentrate its resources in medical centers. Since then, health care has changed dramatically. New organizations—HMOs, health centers, hospital and health care networks, and state agencies—have joined academic medical centers in shaping the careers of health professionals.

Any institution that strives to influence the supply and distribution of health professionals must design programs to work with these organizations. Currently, three programs support consortiums of health providers and training institutions: the Generalist Physician Initiative, Practice Sights, and Partnerships for Training. Systemwide and cross-cutting approaches that move beyond academic medicine in the training and placement of health professionals are the logical way to respond to and influence an increasingly complex health care system.

Improve Distribution of Health Professionals

To increase access to health care requires emphasizing more equitable distribution, as well as an increased supply, of health professionals. Even with increased numbers of generalist and minority physicians, nurse practitioners, and physician assistants, the scarcity of health

Table 2.1 Foundation Fellowship–Faculty Scholar Programs.

Program	Dates	Fellows	Training or Research Focus	Fellows per Year	Length of Awards	Number of Graduates Through 1996	Funding ($ million)
Clinical Nurse Scholars	1982–1991	Nurses	Nursing research, clinical practice and management	9	2 years	62	11
Clinical Scholars	1973–1998	Physicians	Nonbiological health sciences	34 26 RWJF 8 Dept. of Veterans Affairs	2 years	707	85.5
Dental Services Research Scholars	1982–1990	Dentists	Health services	5	2 years	30	5
Faculty Fellowships in Health Care Finance	1985–1994	Health administration faculty	Health care financing	6	1-1/2 years	60	2.5
Family Practice Fellowship	1977–1988	Doctors training to be family practitioners	Family practice	12	2 years	101	11.2
General Pediatric Development	1979–1988	Pediatricians	Developmental pediatrics	12	2 years	111	10.9

Program	Years	Discipline	Goal			
Generalist Physician Faculty Scholars	1993–2004	Physicians	Primary care	15	0	27.8
Health Policy Fellows	1973–1998	Mainly physicians—some nurses and others	Staff work in congress or executive branch	6	133	7
Investigator Awards in Health Policy Research	1994–1999	All disciplines except medicine	Broad health policy	10	1	18
Minority Medical Faculty Development	1984–2000	Minority physicians	Biomedical, clinical health services	12	67	59.4
Nurse Faculty Fellowships	1977–1982	Nurses	Develop nurse-practitioner faculty	20	99	4.8
Scholars in Health Policy Research	1993–1999	Economists, political scientists, sociologists	Multidisciplinary health policy	12	12	12.3

professionals in underserved areas remains critical, and in the current economic and political climate this is likely to worsen. So far, nobody has found the key, if one exists, to overcoming the barriers that discourage health professionals from serving inner city and rural communities. Although it may be, as some commentators have argued, that nothing short of an expanded National Health Service Corps will resolve the problem,[15] the Foundation has made some limited attempts to encourage physicians to practice in underserved areas.

In the 1970s and 1980s, the Foundation addressed the distribution of health professionals as a peripheral part of programs designed to restructure health care delivery, for example, by establishing networks of rural physicians and group practices allied with community hospitals. In the mid-1990s, the Foundation began to address some of the structural and social factors that discourage health care professionals from practicing in rural areas and inner cities: the poor reimbursement, the isolation, and the lack of social amenities and professional opportunities for a spouse that keep health care professionals, no matter how well trained, from serving in rural areas. *Practice Sights,* a five-year program begun in 1993, focuses directly on reducing such barriers. It requires participating health care systems—such as state agencies, academic institutions, and HMOs—to work together. Under this program, health care systems have set up loan forgiveness programs, provided technical assistance in practice management, worked to increase reimbursement rates, and offered other incentives to attract health professionals to inner city and rural practices. A second program, *Reach Out,* is discussed in Chapter One; in the present context we note how it builds on the medical profession's tradition of community service.

Investments in training the health care workforce are necessary, but not sufficient, to increase access by underserved populations to basic health care. As the creation of such programs as Practice Sights and Reach Out suggests, it is important to address the inequitable distribution of health professionals directly.

CONCLUSION

The lessons of the past twenty-four years are both simple and complex. They are simple in demonstrating that an unwavering commitment to improving the health care workforce is required to effect change, or to prepare for it when change comes about for other reasons. The lessons are complex insofar as any single foundation's resources can have only a limited impact in a health care system that is rapidly changing and has many more key players than it did even five years ago.

The challenge for the future is to develop workforce programs that further a vision of universal access within the context of an evolving American health care system where business rather than social values predominate, where incentives to avoid serving sick and vulnerable populations are inherent, and where power has shifted out of the hands of medicine. How institutions, including The Robert Wood Johnson Foundation, meet this challenge will determine the course of health care in the United States.

Endnotes

1. D. Rogers, Robert Wood Johnson Foundation, *Annual Report 1972,* pp. 11–12.
2. N. Kassebaum, "Federal Health Professions Training and Distribution Initiatives: Foundations for a Targeted Approach," *Academic Medicine* 70 (1995), 296–297.
3. National Institutes of Health, *Data Book 1994,* table 20; U.S. Senate Committee on Labor and Human Resources, *Health Professions Education Consolidation and Reauthorization Act of 1995: Report* (1995); R. Rosenblatt and others, "The Effect of Federal Grants on Medical Schools' Production of Primary Care Physicians," *American Journal of Public Health* 83 (1993), 322–328; A. Epstein, "U.S. Teaching Hospitals in the Evolving Health Care System," *JAMA* 273 (1995), 1203–1207.
4. D. Rogers, *Robert Wood Johnson Foundation 1974 Annual Report,* p. 28.
5. R. Fein and J. Rowe, *A Review of the RWJF Clinical Scholars Program,* unpublished (1992), p. 10.
6. J. Evans and C. Royer, *The Robert Wood Johnson Foundation: A Twenty-Year Assessment,* unpublished (1992), p. 10.
7. J. Cantor and others, *Evaluation of the Minority Medical Education Program,* unpublished (1994).
8. K. Bridges and L. Smith, *An Evaluation of the Minority Medical Faculty Development Program of the Robert Wood Johnson Foundation,* unpublished (1995).
9. U. S. Department of Health and Human Services, *Secretary's Commission on Nursing: Final Report* (1988), p. 175.
10. See T. Keenan and others, *Nurses and Doctors: Their Education and Practice* (Cambridge, Mass.: Oelgeschlager, Gunn & Hain, 1992); L. Aiken and

M. Gwyther, "Medicare Funding of Nurse Education," *Journal of the American Medical Association* 273 (1995), 1528–1532; C. Fagin, "The Visible Problems of an 'Invisible' Profession: The Crisis and Challenge for Nursing," in *The Nation's Health* (3rd. ed.), P. Lee and C. Estes, eds. (Boston: Jones & Bartlett, 1990), 190–192; U.S. Dept. of Health and Human Services, *Secretary's Commission on Nursing, Final Report* (1988).

11. The project's final report—written in 1990, when fifty-three scholars had completed training—found that "all of the scholars have remained active in nursing in a leadership role. With three exceptions, all of the scholars are actively involved in academic careers in a major school of nursing." R. de Tornyay, *Final Report on the RWJF Clinical Nurse Scholars Program*, unpublished (1990).

12. R. Bulger, *The Robert Wood Johnson Foundation and Human Resources for Health: Some Observations on the First Twenty Years and Some Proposals for the Next Ten*, unpublished (1992).

13. S. Schroeder, "The Institute of Medicine's Review of the Health Policy Fellowship Programs," in *For the Public Good: Highlights from the Institute of Medicine, 1970–1995* (Washington, D.C.: National Academy Press, 1995), 161–167.

14. Nearly one thousand physicians and two hundred nurses, nurse practitioners, dentists, and physician assistants were trained or received fellowships under the Foundation's programs.

15. R. Reynolds, "Make Health Reform Work. Draft Doctors," *New York Times* (June 1, 1993), p. A17.

Exhibit 2.1. National Workforce Programs, by Date.

Medical School Student Aid Program
- Financial aid for women, minority, and rural medical students
- 1972–1978
- $12,600,000 awarded

Preprofessional Minority Programs
- Enrichment programs for potential medical school candidates
- 1972–1992
- $13,300,000 awarded

Clinical Scholars Program
- Two-year postresidency fellowships in nonbiomedical health sciences for physicians committed to clinical medicine
- 1973–1998
- $85,500,000 authorized
- Currently, thirty-four Clinical Scholars a year are appointed (eight are funded by the Department of Veterans Affairs); 707 scholars completed the program through 1996
- Training is currently offered at the following medical centers: Chicago, Johns Hopkins, Michigan, University of California-Los Angeles, North Carolina, Washington, and Yale. It was offered in the past at University of California-San Francisco and Stanford (a joint program that ran between 1974 and mid–1996), Case Western Reserve (1970–76), Columbia (1975–78), Duke (1969–75; this site was funded under the original program of the Carnegie Corporation and Commonwealth Fund and was not continued when The Robert Wood Johnson Foundation took over the program), George Washington (1975–79), McGill (1970–81), and Pennsylvania (1974–mid–1996)

Dental School Student Aid Program
- Financial aid for women, minority, and rural dental students
- 1973–1978
- $4,000,000 awarded

Health Policy Fellowships Program
- One-year fellowships (three-month orientation organized by the Institute of Medicine followed by a nine-month assignment in Congress or executive branch) in Washington, D.C.
- 1973–1998
- $7,000,000 authorized

Note: Programs with an end date of 1997 and beyond may be extended.

(Exhibit 2.1, continued)

- Six fellowships a year are awarded; 133 fellows completed the program through 1996

National Medical Fellowships

- Financial aid for minority medical students
- 1973–1996
- $10,200,000 authorized

Primary Care Residency Program

- Primary care training for internal medicine and pediatric residents
- 1973–1981
- $10,800,000 awarded to the following medical centers or hospitals: Boston City Hospital, Florida, Harvard, Missouri, Pennsylvania, Rochester, UCLA, UCSF, Washington

Dental Training for Care of the Handicapped

- Development of training programs to improve dental treatment of handicapped patients
- 1974–1979
- $4,900,000 awarded to eleven dental schools: Alabama, UCLA, Columbia, Kentucky, Maryland, Michigan, Minnesota, Nebraska, New York, Tennessee, and Washington

United Student Aid Funds

- Financial assistance
- 1976–1985
- $7,500,000 awarded

Nurse Faculty Fellowship Program

- One-year fellowships to develop core nurse-practitioner faculty
- 1977–1982
- $4,800,000 awarded to four nursing schools: Colorado, Indiana, Maryland, and Rochester
- Twenty fellowships a year were awarded; ninety-nine fellows completed the program

Primary Care Training for Emergency Nurses

- Certificate training in primary care for nursing staff of rural hospitals
- 1977–1982
- $1,900,000 awarded to six hospital training sites

Family Practice Faculty Fellowships Program

- Two-year postresidency fellowships in family practice for physicians planning academic careers
- 1978–1988

- $11,200,000 awarded. Five medical centers offered fellowship training initially: Case Western Reserve, Iowa, Missouri-Columbia, Utah, and Washington-Seattle. It was later reduced to three (Washington-Seattle, Missouri-Columbia, and Case Western Reserve)
- Twelve fellowships a year were awarded; 101 fellows completed the program

General Pediatric Academic Development Program
- Two-year fellowships to train future pediatric faculty in general pediatrics
- 1979–1988
- $10,900,000 awarded to six academic medical centers: Duke, Johns Hopkins, Pennsylvania, Rochester, Stanford, and Yale
- Twelve fellowships a year were awarded; 111 pediatricians completed the program

Clinical Nurse Scholars Program
- Two-year scholarships to develop a core nursing faculty skilled in research, clinical practice, and management
- 1982–1991
- $11,000,000 awarded for training at three sites: Pennsylvania, Rochester, and UCSF
- Nine scholarships a year were awarded; sixty-two scholars completed the program

Dental Services Research Scholars Program
- Two-year fellowships to train dental faculty in nonclinical health sciences and health services
- 1982–1990
- $5,000,000 awarded for training at two sites (Harvard and UCLA)
- Five scholarships a year were awarded; thirty scholars completed the program

Minority Medical Faculty Development Program
- Four-year postdoctoral research fellowships for minority physicians committed to careers in academic medicine
- 1984–2000
- $59,400,000 authorized
- Currently, twelve fellowships a year are awarded; sixty-seven fellows completed the program through 1996

Faculty Fellowships in Health Care Finance
- Thirty-month fellowships—three-month (later changed to four) orientation at The Johns Hopkins University, followed by a nine-month (later changed to eight) assignment to a health care financing organization and up to eighteen months' research

(Exhibit 2.1, continued)

- 1985–1994
- $2,500,000 awarded
- Six fellowships a year were awarded; sixty fellows completed the program

Minority Medical Education Program

- Six-week summer program for minority college students considering medical school
- 1988–1999
- $15,300,000 authorized. As of 1996, eight sites offer training: Alabama, Baylor, Case Western Reserve, Chicago Consortium led by Rush University, United Negro College Fund (Fisk University/Vanderbilt), Virginia, Western Consortium led by the University of Washington School of Medicine, and Yale. The Illinois Institute of Technology was a site between 1988 and 1995.
- 125 students a year are selected per site; 5,500 students have completed the program through 1996

Strengthening Hospital Nursing: A Program to Improve Patient Care

- Grants to hospitals to improve patient care by restructuring services around the nursing staff
- 1989–1995
- A $26.8 million joint program with the Pew Charitable Trusts. RWJF awarded $16,500,000 for twenty planning grants, fifteen phase one implementation grants, and fourteen phase two implementation grants

Nursing Services Manpower Development Program

- Four-year grants, on average, to institutions to attract more minorities and others (older women, single mothers) to nursing careers and to overcome the barriers to their entering the profession
- 1989–1994
- $3,200,000 awarded to institutions in seven states: California, Illinois, Iowa, Indiana, New York, Pennsylvania, and Texas

Generalist Physician Initiative

- Grants to academic medical centers, in collaboration with HMOs, state governments, private insurers, hospitals, and community health centers, to increase the number of general internists, general pediatricians, and family practitioners
- 1991–2000
- $32,700,000 authorized planning grants were awarded to eighteen medical centers or consortiums in 1992; of these, fourteen received implementation grants: Boston, Case Western Reserve, Dartmouth, East Carolina, Hahnemann, Massachusetts, Georgia, Nevada, New Mexico, New York Medical College, Pennsylvania State, Texas-Galveston, SUNY/Buffalo, Virginia

Generalist Physician Faculty Scholars Program
- Four-year grants to medical school faculty to conduct research related to primary care
- 1993–2004
- $27,800,000 authorized
- Fifteen scholars a year are selected

Generalist Provider Research Initiative
- Research on generalist/specialist mix and distribution and to evaluate the Foundation's generalist programs in a larger context
- 1993–1998
- $3,000,000 authorized

Ladders in Nursing Careers (National Replication)
- National replication of program developed in 1988 by the Greater New York Hospital Foundation. Grants to hospital associations to assist minority and other disadvantaged (e.g., single parents) housekeeping staff, nurses' aides, and nurses to advance their careers.
- 1993–1997
- $4,900,000 authorized. Through the end of 1995, awards were made to hospital associations in nine states: Georgia, Iowa, Maryland, Minnesota, North Dakota, Ohio, Rhode Island, South Carolina, and Texas

Scholars in Health Policy Research
- Two-year postdoctoral fellowships to economists, political scientists, and sociologists to conduct health care research
- 1993–1999
- $12,300,000 authorized
- Twelve scholars a year are selected

Investigator Awards in Health Policy Research
- Three years' salary support for outstanding young researchers or eminent senior scholars to pursue health care research
- 1994–1999
- $18,000,000 authorized
- Ten investigators are selected each year

Partnerships for Training: Regional Education Systems for Nurse Practitioners, Certified Nurse-Midwives, and Physician Assistants
- Support of innovative and collaborative education models for training nurse practitioners, certified nurse-midwives, and physician assistants in their own communities
- 1995–2001
- $14,000,000 authorized
- Planning grants were made to organizations in twelve states: Arkansas,

(Exhibit 2.1, continued)

California, Colorado, Idaho, Illinois, Michigan, Minnesota, New Mexico, New York, North Carolina, Pennsylvania, and Wisconsin

Colleagues in Caring: Regional Collaboratives for Nursing Workforce Development

- Grants to regional consortiums of nursing schools, hospitals, and nursing service providers and associations to assess and meet the nursing needs in the region
- 1996–1999
- $4,000,000 authorized

Project 3000 by 2000: Health Professions Partnership Initiative

- Grants to academic medical centers, working in partnership with local schools, colleges, and community organizations, to attract minority high school students to health professions and to nurture their interest
- 1996–2001
- $5,000,000 authorized for grants to the following medical centers: Connecticut, Georgia, Louisville, Massachusetts, Nebraska, North Carolina, Oregon, Pennsylvania/Hahnemann, South Carolina, and Wisconsin-Madison. Up to five additional sites will be selected in the future.

~ A Review of the National Access-to-Care Surveys

Marc L. Berk
Claudia L. Schur

Editors' Introduction

Chapter Three documents the strategies used over time by Foundation grantees tracking access to health care among Americans. The four national surveys of access to care that are discussed represent the Foundation's flagship investment in analysis related to problems of access. One goal of these surveys has been to gain an understanding of the extent and nature of the problem. An even more important goal has been to focus attention on the problems faced by individuals who cannot get basic health care services.

The chapter avoids reporting findings or trends from the surveys, which have been published in a large number of academic papers, Foundation reports, and monographs. Instead, the chapter examines the evolution of the surveys and the shifting aims and priorities over the past twenty years. It highlights the challenges survey researchers face in studying access to health care, and it explains how approaches to measuring access have also evolved over the past two decades.

This chapter introduces readers to the logic of the Foundation's efforts in this area. It offers a guide to interpreting access-to-care research and puts the surveys supported by the Foundation into the context of other data-collection efforts that have measured service use, access, and expenditures on health care over the years.

The authors, Marc L. Berk and Claudia L. Schur, are the director and deputy director, respectively, of the Center for Health Affairs at Project HOPE. They have directed the Foundation's most recent access-to-care survey and are publishing a series of papers and reports on findings from the 1994 survey. Meanwhile, fieldwork on the latest Foundation-supported access survey was completed as this book was being printed. The 1997 approach to measuring access allows for assessments of access problems in twelve distinct communities along with the nation as a whole. The community focus of the newest survey reflects the growing importance of understanding how emerging market dynamics—which vary from community to community—affect access to care among vulnerable populations.

E ven after the extensive debate over the reform of the health care system in the early 1990s, the basic issue of universal health care as a fundamental right of Americans remains unresolved among our nation's leaders and among our citizens. Media reports about people who lack access to medical care may push emotional buttons—the elderly man left unattended for hours in an emergency room, say, or the poor pregnant woman who receives no medical attention until she goes into premature labor and delivers a one-and-a-half-pound infant—but only occasionally do they have an impact on public policy. It has long been known that what policy makers need is not anecdotal evidence like this but hard, reliable information on access to medical care.

In a 1980 foreword to the classic book on access to care, David Rogers and Linda Aiken of The Robert Wood Johnson Foundation wrote of the lack of availability of such information:

> Despite the large efforts made during the preceding decade to improve medical care for Americans, there was startlingly little solid information on the extent of the remaining access problem, on who was having difficulty obtaining medical care, or on whether the multitude of programs initiated during the 1960s had been successful. The studies then available were primarily head counts on the numbers of doctors within geographic areas, or simply records on mortality and morbidity within different regions. Although these statistics had some usefulness for overall planning, they did not provide the kind of information needed to design targeted strategies for getting underserved people better health and medical care.[1]

Acknowledging the necessity of having objective, systematic, and scientific data available for policy making, the Foundation launched its first national survey of access to care in 1976.

The survey followed a number of other efforts (Table 3.1) aimed at systematically measuring access to and expenditures on health care for population subgroups and for the nation as a whole.[2] In the early 1930s, the Falk Commission on the Costs of Medical Care—an independent group of representatives from organized medicine, the government, academic social science, and the hospital and insurance

Table 3.1 Selected National Health Surveys.

Year	Survey	Sponsor	Primary Focus
Early 1930s	Falk Commission on the Costs of Medical Care	Independent representatives from private and public sectors	National health care expenditure estimates
1953–54	Costs of Medical Care of Two Cities: Boston and Birmingham	Center for Health Administration Studies, University of Chicago	Health care costs and insurance status
1953 and periodically through 1975	Medical Care Costs and Voluntary Health Insurance	Center for Health Administration Studies, University of Chicago	Measure public's use of medical services and methods of payment
1955	Attitudes, Information, and Customary Behavior in Health Matters	Center for Health Administration Studies, University of Chicago	How people learn about health conditions and treatments
1957 and annually thereafter	National Health Interview Survey	National Center for Health Statistics	Statistics on disease, injury, impairment, disability, etc.
1963 and 1970	Health Care Use and Expenditure Survey	Center for Health Administration Studies, University of Chicago*	Effects of government financing on use and expenditures; distributional implications
1977	National Medical Care Expenditure Survey	National Center for Health Services Research and National Center for Health Statistics	National use and expenditure estimates; general health policy/financing research
1980	National Medical Care Utilization and Expenditure Survey	National Center for Health Statistics	National use and expenditure estimates; general health policy/financing research
1987	National Medical Expenditure Survey	Agency for Health Care Policy and Research	National use and expenditure estimates; general health policy/financing research
1996 and annually thereafter	Medical Expenditure Panel Survey	Agency for Health Care Policy and Research	National use and expenditure estimates; general health policy/financing research

* The 1970 study was funded by the National Center for Health Services Research.

industries—sponsored the first survey intended to produce estimates of national health care expenditures. During the next several decades, there were sporadic, small-scale, health-related survey efforts, but none were national in scope; nor were they focused primarily on health expenditures or access to care.

With legislators and health care professionals demanding information to use in making policy decisions, Public Law 652 was passed in 1956 to authorize the regular collection of health-related data "to produce statistics on disease, injury, impairment, disability, and related topics on a uniform basis for the nation as a whole." This survey was later renamed the National Health Interview Survey (NHIS), and it has been conducted annually since 1957. Until recent years, its primary emphasis was on collecting health status information and, to a lesser degree, the use of services. Only in the past decade has a major focus been on insurance status and other measures of access to care.

The next entry in the progression of national health surveys was the 1963 Health Care Use and Expenditure Survey, conducted by the Center for Health Administration Studies at the University of Chicago. It was followed by a 1970 survey of the same name and, subsequently, two expenditure surveys sponsored by the federal government (the 1977 National Medical Care Expenditure Survey and the 1987 National Medical Expenditure Survey). In contrast to the NHIS, these four surveys were designed to provide data that would help policy makers understand the effects of government financing programs on the use of services and expenditures, assess the distributional implications of programs and the availability of health care services, and identify and evaluate problems in access to care for different population subgroups.

The surveys conducted after 1965 and into the 1970s attempted to measure changes in access brought about by major governmental expansion into health care: the Medicare and Medicaid programs. As federal expenditures climbed and government became a major purchaser of health care, costs became the primary focus and access was relegated to a secondary consideration. The emphasis on cost necessitated several design changes between the 1970 Health Care Use and Expenditure Survey and the 1977 National Medical Care Expenditure Survey. Multiple interviews and shorter recall periods—requiring respondents to remember events over a three- to four-month period rather than a year—facilitated the collection of detailed cost and payment data. In addition, components were added to verify the charge and use data of medical providers and to obtain information from health insurers on health benefits not available from the household; these numbers were used to support estimates of national health care expenditures and sources of payment by a variety of population subgroups.

When the first Robert Wood Johnson Foundation access survey was undertaken in 1976, however, little of this groundwork had been laid. In addition to asserting the need for hard empirical evidence, the Foundation, along with the National Center for Health Services Research, supported what remains the seminal work in establishing well-defined and widely accepted means of measuring access to care. These measures of access were developed by Ron Andersen and Lu Ann Aday as part of a framework for studying access to health care. The measures were tested on the 1976 access-to-care survey. While this was the fifth in a series of health care surveys undertaken by the University of Chicago, the first four emphasized families' health care experiences and costs, whereas the 1976 survey concerned individuals' access to the health care system. A major focus of the study, as voiced by the Foundation, was to "carefully describe the exact subgroups of our population who continue to have difficulty in getting medical care." Thus, there were twin themes of measuring access and charting the equity of access across different population subgroups.

This original framework focused on four major types of indicators:

- Characteristics of the health care delivery system
- Characteristics of the population at risk
- Utilization of health care services
- Consumer satisfaction

The first two were intended to reflect *potential* access to medical care, while the last two indicators measure *realized* access. Behind this framework was the assumption that public policy could be used to affect realized access through changes in potential access. Suppose, for example, that policy makers learn that people who live in areas with few health professionals have fewer health care visits than those who live in areas where health care providers are plentiful. Within the Aday-Andersen framework, the number of health care visits made by different population subgroups is an indicator of realized access; in order to increase the number of visits for those in specific geographic areas, policy makers might try to increase the supply of health care providers in those areas. So, too, altering a part of the health care delivery system, for example, reorganizing the financing and delivery of services, might affect realized access to care.

This broad framework has supported much of the policy research related to access to care over the last twenty years. During this period, access to a wide range of services has improved, and for substantial portions of the population. Much of the overall improvement in the health status of Americans is attributable to increased access to care: more widespread use of Pap smears and pelvic exams has contributed to a decline in mortality from cervical cancer, and the expansion of 911 emergency medical systems has increased survival from out-of-hospital cardiac arrest, stroke, and trauma.

CHANGES IN APPROACHES TO MEASURING ACCESS

The original framework developed by Aday and Andersen for studying access to care remains in wide use today. Health services researchers continue to be concerned about the organization of health care systems and the availability of resources; about how personal characteristics affect interactions with the health care system; about the level of use of health care services; and about consumers' satisfaction with their care. Within these broad categories, however, emphases have shifted over time, and there has been a move toward measuring the effects of access on health outcomes.

The themes explored in the four Foundation-supported access surveys (1976, 1982, 1986, and 1994; see Table 3.2) have evolved to reflect society's most pressing problems. The methodological approaches have varied in keeping with goals, constraints on resources, and changes in the way data are collected. The first of the surveys relied on in-person interviews with eight thousand people. A number of groups were oversampled: persons with episodes of illness, nonurban Southern blacks, and Hispanics living in the Southwest. Substantively, the survey emphasized attributes of the respondents' usual source of care, including convenience and consumer satisfaction, illness-related symptoms, and the use of health care services.

While the study originally intended to provide baseline data for an evaluation of a specific health initiative, the larger goal was to develop empirical indicators of access that could be used to monitor changes

Table 3.2 Overview of the Robert Wood Johnson Foundation National Access-to-Care Surveys: 1976, 1982, 1986, and 1994.

Year	Institution	Sample Size	Interview Mode	Oversampled Groups	Selected Major Findings	Design Issues
1976	Center for Health Administration Studies, University of Chicago	7,787	In person	■ Individuals with episodes of illness ■ Non-SMSA Southern blacks ■ Hispanics in the Southwestern United States	■ Percent with usual source of care (USOC) up for elderly and poor; uninsured remain most likely to have no USOC. ■ Access worse (e.g., longer travel times and lower rates of insurance coverage) among farm dwellers, residents of the South—particularly non-urban Southern blacks—and Hispanics in Southwest. ■ Hospital and physician services obtained according to illness levels. Dental care more dependent on social structural variables and family resources and less on need. ■ People generally satisfied with care; highest levels of dissatisfaction with out-of-pocket medical care costs and waiting times in clinics and physician offices.	

| 1982 | Center for Health Administration Studies, University of Chicago | 6,610 | Telephone | Individuals with family incomes below 150% of poverty | • Poor, minorities, central city, and farm residents mostly maintained or improved with respect to having a USOC or using hospital, physician, and preventive services.
• Access problems continue for disadvantaged groups with respect to site of USOC, waiting times for care, and levels of satisfaction with care. Uninsured most consistently disadvantaged in terms of access indicators.
• Even after adjustment for need and other factors, the uninsured and those without a USOC have lower rates of hospitalization and lower rates of use of adult preventive services.
• Of families with a seriously or chronically ill family member, 22% reported a major financial problem as a result. Most likely to report major financial problems were the uninsured (52%), poor nonwhites (50%), blacks (40%), Hispanics (39%), and people with public insurance only (36%). | • Potential undercount of uninsured and other vulnerable populations due to reliance on telephone interviews. |

Table 3.2, continued

Year	Institution	Sample Size	Interview Mode	Oversampled Groups	Selected Major Findings	Design Issues
1986	Institute for Social Sciences Research, University of California, Los Angeles	10,130	Telephone	■ Individuals with chronic and serious illnesses	■ Overall use of medical care (in terms of hospital admissions and physician visits) declined. Access to physician care for individuals who were poor, black, or uninsured decreased between 1982 and 1986, particularly for those in poor health. ■ Disadvantaged groups (including blacks, Hispanics, and the uninsured) continue to receive less hospital care than might be appropriate given their higher rate of ill health. ■ The long-standing gap in receipt of medical care between rural and urban residents appears to have been eliminated. ■ Most Americans continue to be highly satisfied with their physician and inpatient hospital care.	■ Sole reliance on telephone interviewing led to undercount of uninsured. ■ Small number of persons denied care resulted in cell size too small for much analysis.

| 1994 | Project HOPE Center for Health Affairs | 7,562 | Mixed mode: telephone, with in-person interviews for persons with no phones or hearing impaired | Individuals with poor access or specific health conditions, as identified through an existing national probability survey | ■ Proportion of persons reporting inability to obtain needed medical/surgical care has remained relatively constant since 1982, at about 6% of the population.

■ Using more inclusive definition of health care needs (including medical/surgical care, dental care, prescription drugs, eyeglasses, and mental health care), 16.1% of respondents (more than 41 million Americans) were unable to obtain at least one service they believed they needed.

■ For each service, Medicaid enrollees were half as likely to report problems as uninsured and twice as likely as privately insured.

■ HMO enrollees had more physician visits than persons in traditional plans but are more likely to report unmet medical need. | ■ Undercount of uninsured reduced substantially but not eliminated due to continued reliance on telephone for most interviews |

in the study population. Such data could also inform policy makers about the population subgroups who faced the greatest barriers to access, and the data could provide a basis for analyzing how well existing programs succeeded in improving access.

The 1982 survey continued this general approach, focusing on whether the previous trends for the major indicators of access were continuing, which groups appeared to have the greatest problems, and the severity of certain problems that might be exacerbated by the political and economic climate.[3] Emphasis on this latter objective was facilitated through an oversample of families with incomes below 150 percent of the federal poverty level. Attention continued to be focused on the usual source of care (including the site of care and waiting times); the use of hospital, physician, and preventive services; and insurance coverage or eligibility for public programs. A new area of concern—prompted by increasing health care cost consciousness combined with an economic recession—emphasized barriers encountered in obtaining care for a family member with a serious illness. Methodologically, the 1982 survey undertook one of the first highly visible applications of random-digit dialing techniques, using telephone interviews to reach its approximately sixty-six hundred respondents at a cost substantially lower than that of in-person interviews.

In their analysis of survey data, Aday, Andersen, and Gretchen Fleming wrote of "the special access problems created by long-term chronic illness,"[4] suggesting that even people with usually adequate third-party coverage were unable to pay for the long-term health care needs posed by chronic illness. With these findings in mind, the 1986 survey (consisting of telephone interviews with approximately ten thousand people) included an oversample of Americans with chronic and serious illness. The content of the survey continued to focus on the availability of a usual source of care; use of services; self-reports of health status, including the presence of serious health conditions; problems in paying for care; and satisfaction. In contrast to the findings from the two earlier surveys, results from 1986 indicated an overall decline in the use of medical care and increasing disparities in the use of services between the American mainstream and members of vulnerable population subgroups such as the poor, the uninsured, and minorities.[5]

Although a secondary goal of the 1994 survey was to monitor trends in access, the Foundation was primarily interested in taking a fresh look at both the methodology and the policy objectives of the survey. We were particularly interested in increasing the survey's analytic capabilities (larger sample sizes of populations of interest) without increasing data collection costs.

This was accomplished with a methodological approach employed in other data-collection efforts but never before for an access survey: using the National Health Interview Survey to target respondents who reported access problems. Some of these individuals were contacted for a follow-up interview that focused additional attention on their problems in gaining access to health care. Most interviews were conducted by telephone (in order to keep costs down); these were supplemented with in-person interviews of people without telephones or people who were functionally unable to be interviewed by telephone. The 1994 survey comprised three components: (1) a national probability sample, (2) a sample of persons who reported access barriers or who met other specific criteria suggesting low access to care, and (3) a sample of persons with one of two specific chronic conditions for which well-accepted standards of care exist.

Given the Foundation's continued interest in the organization of medical care and its effect on access, data on the usual source of care were collected, although it was deemphasized somewhat. The survey also examined predisposing characteristics, including age, race, sex, and attitudes about the efficacy of medicine. The ability to assess the role of health status in the use of services was emphasized through a new symptom-response sequence developed with separate funding from the Foundation. A focus on financial barriers to care was expanded through a series of questions on paid sick leave from work.

Over the last two decades, seemingly small changes in the emphasis of the access surveys are part of a larger pattern in the study of access to health care. While it remains important to analyze changes over time, social science research cannot be held hostage to old ideas. It must adapt to changing circumstances, even though comparability of particular questions over time is sacrificed. Researchers have become increasingly sophisticated in their approach to data collection. They are better able to target populations of interest and select appropriate methods to reach them. They have adopted a healthy skepticism about soliciting the opinions of our health care consumers ("Don't tell us what you think; let us observe what you do"). Faced with increasing budgetary pressures, our society is reluctant to increase access for its own sake. Instead, it demands to know how increases in resources and in the use of health care services affect health outcomes.

New Data Collection Strategies

The most recent survey went beyond counting the instances in which people felt that they could not get care; it provided a context giving their reason for seeking care. In addition, the survey tracked the condition for which they sought care, whether they were eventually treated, and how they felt their health was affected by the treatment or lack of treatment.

Although collection of in-depth information on the circumstances surrounding unmet need was motivated by policy considerations, it was made possible by more sophisticated data-collection methods than had been previously used. In any nationally representative sample, only a small number of the respondents encounter serious access problems, so having a sufficient number of "cases" for analytic purposes is difficult. Increasing the sample size is costly and inefficient; for every person with access problems added to the sample, many other persons with no problems are added, and data collection costs rise prohibitively.

To overcome this problem, the 1994 survey used the National Health Interview Survey as a giant screener to identify people having low access. These people fell into one of the following categories:

- Those who reported unmet need for medical care or surgery

- Those who reported a hospital emergency room as their usual source of care

- Those who reported being in fair or poor health but who had not seen a physician in the past year

- Those who reported having delayed care for financial reasons

With 120,000 respondents to the NHIS annually, we were able to select people who reported access problems in the NHIS for follow-up interviews, thereby increasing the sample size in a cost-efficient manner and concentrating interview time on those with the most serious access problems.

Measuring Behavior Versus Opinions

The public opinion polls have been awash in news of consumer dissatisfaction with the health care system; political careers have been made and lost gambling on just how widespread consumer dissatisfaction is, and pundits argue over the interpretation of the polling results. While the majority of people report dissatisfaction with the general state of health care, as individuals they are quite satisfied with the care they receive.[6] This presents something of an anomaly for policy makers: do they attempt to fix the health care system about which people complain or do they protect the status quo because most individuals are happy with their own care? As one of the present authors noted in a recent *Health Affairs* commentary, "the problem is not in the polls themselves, but rather in the unrealistic expectations that we have placed on the polling process. Polls are only one predictor of how people are likely to behave and, indeed, polls are probably not the most accurate."[7]

It is better, instead, to find out what people do rather than what they say. With the growing role of economics in the study of health policy, analysts are using the methods of what economists call "revealed preference": deducing an individual's preferences from observed choices or behavior. Thus, researchers collect data on people's health insurance coverage, their demographic characteristics and health status, and their medical care use and expenditures, and they make inferences about the underlying relationships and causal factors. In fact, from the perspective of trying to understand and explain why and how individuals use health care, opinion questions have never proved to be particularly good predictors of health care use.

Researchers have also begun to think more objectively about what can be learned from questions about satisfaction. Responses to these questions may tell more about the site of care or the expectations of the patient than about the quality of the care delivered. Some differences in satisfaction have been traced to variations in the supply of health resources; in these cases, individuals are responding to different circumstances surrounding the delivery of care. In reviewing findings on satisfaction over time, Howard Freeman and Martin Shapiro remark that "it is a reasonable hypothesis that the ambiance of physicians' offices and the validation of parking receipts may be equally as strong determinants of satisfaction as correct diagnoses and appropriate treatment."[8]

Thus, within the access surveys themselves, there has been a moderate deemphasis on subjective measures of access such as satisfaction with care and overall views about the American medical system, and an increasing emphasis on observable behavior. Certain questions

were included in the 1994 survey to discover attitudes toward the efficacy of medicine; others elicited reactions to health care reform. In
addition, the 1994 survey included a sequence in which respondents
were asked whether they ever experienced a particular symptom and,
if so, whether they sought medical care. With independent ratings of
the seriousness of the symptoms from physicians, a more objective
assessment could be made of care-seeking behavior.

Fine-Tuning Questions Versus Maintaining Continuity

Researchers who monitor trends are always faced with a dilemma: how
to improve a survey and still make it comparable to surveys that have
been done in the past? As more resources are invested in gathering
data with which to make health policy decisions, more is learned
about the difficulty of gathering *reliable* data. Seemingly small changes
in survey design—minor alterations to the way the respondents are
chosen, revisions in the wording of a question, and even changes in
the ways interviewers are trained—can fundamentally affect the
responses people give.

The designers of the Foundation-supported access surveys, as well
as the designers of other major health surveys, must decide whether
it is more important to measure changes over time or to obtain the
most accurate estimate possible of how things stand at a single point
in time. An example of this type of decision and how it affects analysts' ability to provide policy-relevant information is a change in the
Current Population Survey (CPS), which, among other things, is used
to make estimates of health insurance coverage and, in particular, to
monitor growth or decline in the size of the uninsured population. In
the late 1980s, the issue of whether CPS estimates of the uninsured
population were "annual" or "point-in-time" was the subject of some
controversy.[9] Because of the attention focused on the issue, wording
changes were made; while these may have increased the reliability of
the estimates since 1989, they have made the longitudinal study of patterns of coverage more difficult. To avoid these difficulties, many surveys, such as the National Health Interview Survey, place emphasis on
maintaining continuity and make changes only where there is strong
evidence that the current procedure is not working well; even then,
changes are closely monitored to ensure the reliability of data.

When the 1994 access survey was designed, eight years had elapsed since the last survey. We convened a technical advisory panel of leading experts in survey methods and health policy. There was a consensus that while monitoring trends in access to care was important, preserving the ability to measure such trends should not come at the expense of accurately enumerating the problems in access to care that were being experienced in the 1990s. Accordingly, when better ways were found to ask questions, or to select our sample, we used them, even though doing so complicated our ability to do trend analysis.

Two examples illustrate this point. Previous access surveys used symptom/response questions to measure whether people are receiving care for specific symptoms they have experienced. The Foundation had already invested considerable resources to improve symptom/response questions. In the course of developing the 1994 survey, a greater effort was made to develop lists of symptoms for which there was a strong medical consensus about appropriate medical care. These questions (developed by Shapiro and Freeman) were substituted for those used previously. While this change makes comparisons with earlier surveys more difficult, it does provide a more valid indicator of differences in obtaining medical care across population subgroups.

A second example is our use of in-person interviews. The 1982 and 1986 access surveys used telephone interviews exclusively. Some studies have indicated that telephone surveys may exclude poor or disadvantaged people who do not have a telephone; these people are disproportionately likely to have access problems. In order to reduce the bias that might be associated with relying solely on telephone interviews, the 1994 survey conducted in-person interviews with those who had no phone or who had a disability that prevented them from using a telephone.

Broadening the Definitions of Financial Barriers

"Coming full circle" might best describe the evolution of the four access surveys' outlook on financial barriers to care. Health services researchers often make a distinction between financial factors that inhibit access (such as insurance coverage and income) and cultural or attitudinal factors (such as inability to speak English or lack of trust in physicians). While the first survey oversampled members of disadvantaged groups (Southern blacks and Hispanics in the Southwest), the focus was not primarily on their cultural differences but on their economic differences, and how the latter disparity influenced the use of medical care.

Most research indicates that financial barriers to care are better predictors of the use of services than variables that reflect attitudes about the delivery or the efficacy of medicine, or even indicators of cultural or language differences. Yet we wanted to account fully for all possible dimensions of access: a lack of health insurance and low income are probably the most important financial barriers faced by those seeking services, but we hoped to measure other economic obstacles to care. For example, an employee may have good health insurance but not have adequate sick leave to visit a doctor without loss of pay. Similarly, a child might be covered under a parent's insurance policy, but the parent cannot afford to take time off from work without financial consequences. Thus, we asked a series of questions about sick leave as well as the travel cost associated with seeking medical care.

In developing these questions, we wanted to get a better idea of the *real* consequences of taking time off from work. Many employers do not officially allow employees to take time off from work to care for sick children, for example, but in practice supervisors may grant such leave when it is requested. Conversely, although an employee may have a large bank of sick leave, absence from the office can adversely affect how he or she is evaluated or compensated. The 1994 access survey asks questions specifically designed to find out about informal mechanisms that might have financial consequences for those seeking care.

Moving Toward Need-Based Measures of Access

An important factor influencing the use of health services is the need for medical care, which the access surveys have attempted to measure in a variety of ways. Without reviewing medical records, however, measuring need remains a tricky endeavor; some people are simply not very good at reporting on their health in a way that allows for systematic comparisons with what other people have reported. With this rather substantial caveat in mind, the most often-used measure of health is a self-reported health status measure with four possible levels: excellent, good, fair, or poor.

In order to better study those with the highest level of need for health care services, both the 1976 and the 1986 surveys oversampled sick people. The 1976 survey placed special emphasis on people with episodes of illness, while adults and children with chronic conditions or severe illnesses were overrepresented in the 1986 study. In the 1994 survey, with the added power provided by the NHIS, two specific chronic conditions were selected for special investigation: asthma and ischemic heart disease. People who reported having either of these conditions in the NHIS were selected for follow-up interviews.

Focusing on specific health conditions allows analysts to establish a baseline of need and devote attention to assessing differences in access among population subgroups. The two chronic conditions were chosen with the following factors in mind: high incidence rates to provide sufficient numbers of cases for analysis; empirical evidence suggesting that household respondents can self-report accurately; and well-accepted standards for care of the conditions. For each of the conditions, a physician helped design questions to elicit from survey respondents a brief natural history of the disease, past treatment, symptoms, and functional status. Comparison across population subgroups in terms of treatment and health care use will be used to evaluate access to care.

Adapting to Changing Health Delivery Systems and Political Context

The central role of the federal government in the financing of health care spurred the growth of health services research as we know it today. With the advent of the Medicare and Medicaid programs in the 1960s came the imperative to study their impact—a major thrust of research on access to care in the early 1970s was assessing the changes brought about by these programs—and to prepare for national health insurance.

But the moment passed, and in the 1980s the nation's attention turned to supply-side economics and tax cutting. The health care sector was faced with the persistence of escalating health care costs and the intransigence of the various health care players in being the first to change behavior. There was a widespread realization as well that nudging coinsurance rates and deductibles had little effect on the cost of health care. The real players in the health care system were the providers, and it was their behavior that needed to be modified. The move in 1983 from cost-based hospital reimbursement under Medicare to paying a fixed amount based on diagnosis was the beginning of the evolution toward altering financial incentives for providers.

Then came the effort in the 1990s to reform the nation's health care system. By the time the reform effort ended, it had become increasingly clear that changes in the health care system do not come exclusively—or even, perhaps, primarily—from policy makers at the national level. The delivery of health care has been changing at a mind-altering pace ever since.

Health care experts and policy makers must understand not only these changes but also the way they affect how researchers formulate questions and collect data. It is no longer sufficient to ask respondents if they are covered by a private insurance policy; in order to understand their use of health care, we must attempt to ascertain whether it is a health maintenance organization or a preferred provider organization, whether the physician is paid on a fee-for-service or a capitated basis, and so on. And we must deal with analytic complexities, imposed not only by the myriad insurance arrangements but also by the inability of both consumers and providers to understand their arrangements. We may hypothesize, for instance, that a specific payment arrangement (for example, a salary bonus to physicians at the end of the year if expenditures on treatment have been lower than expected) may influence the way in which physicians prescribe care. Yet does it make sense to even study this hypothesis when recent studies show that many physicians do not understand how their treatment decisions affect their pay? If a physician doesn't know that he or she is subject to a salary withhold, does it affect how he or she provides care?

At the same time, the political climate continues to change—with dramatic potential for altering access to care under public programs. Every new Congress has its own views on what to do with the federally sponsored programs that make up the safety net. In order to monitor changes and develop an understanding of the effects of local public programs on access to care, the 1994 survey developed a methodology for studying the role of community-based and local health programs in promoting access. By gathering information about county-based and other local health care programs in the communities from which we drew respondents, it is possible to investigate the effect of these programs on access to care.

LESSONS LEARNED ABOUT
TRENDS IN ACCESS

Although much of what we learn when we study access to health care is disheartening, this may be a glass-is-half-empty phenomenon. By and large, most studies of access find that the majority of Americans are able to obtain the health care they need and are satisfied with it. One of the first findings from the 1994 access survey, published in *Health Affairs,* noted that "approximately 6 percent of Americans are unable to obtain the medical care or surgical care they believe they need."[10] This was similar to the proportion of persons reporting unmet need in both the 1982 and 1986 surveys, showing a surprising constancy over time. Looking at the number from the glass-is-half-full perspective, in each of the survey years 94 percent of those surveyed were essentially saying that they had no trouble getting the medical or surgical care they needed. For Americans as a whole, physician visit rates—in particular, the proportion of persons who are able to get into the system for at least one visit—have also been relatively steady over time, while hospitalization rates have tended slightly downward, in part because of changes in the financial incentives facing those institutions. A clear majority of Americans queried in public opinion polls express satisfaction with their own health care; this is true for persons in traditional fee-for-service arrangements as well as those in HMOs or other managed care plans.

There is some evidence that certain types of health care use may be declining. Preliminary trend estimates from the access-to-care surveys (part of ongoing analyses) indicate that, on a per capita basis, the number of physician visits is declining somewhat. It should be stressed that this may be "just what the doctor ordered"—that the focus should not be on maintaining a given number of visits but on the appropriateness of care. In an increasingly managed care environment, fewer visits may mean that costs are under control and that incentives to provide increasing amounts of care have been neutralized. This notion applies to the downturn in hospital admission rates as well. Researchers are increasingly making the distinction between overall hospitalizations and those for a special class of conditions sensitive to ambulatory care: if individuals receive appropriate ambulatory treatment for the condition, they should not require hospitalization. In examining this specific class of conditions, we can more clearly assess whether changes in the use of services are indicative of an access problem.

Looking beyond outpatient and hospital inpatient services, we observe phenomena that remind us, as researchers, to be ever vigilant in defining *access to care*. Some of the greatest barriers to care are registered when the definition of health care includes a wider range of services, such as dental care and eyeglasses. Casting the net wider, 16.1 percent of respondents to the 1994 access survey—representing more than forty-one million people—were unable to obtain at least one service they believed they needed. This is substantially larger than the 6 percent figure cited above. Since there are no comparison data about these other services from past surveys, the finding by itself provides no evidence as to whether access to care has either improved or deteriorated. Yet it calls attention to the need to be cautious in defining access. As is true with all research, the answer one gets depends on the question asked. While prescription drugs and dental care consume far less of the health care dollar than inpatient services or ambulatory physician services, they are critical for the nation's health, have serious implications for quality of life, and should be examined more systematically.

In addition to traditional services, alternative medicine is seen as important to health for an increasing number of people. Estimates from the 1994 survey indicate that nearly 10 percent of the U.S. population saw a professional in 1994 for at least one of the following four therapies: chiropractic, relaxation techniques, therapeutic massage, or acupuncture. Some may argue, perhaps justifiably, that insuring access to therapeutic massage is not part of the nation's health policy agenda, but the use of these services and their health-related outcomes should be monitored.

Since their inception, the access-to-care surveys have focused not only on the level of access achieved by the majority but also on equity in access across population subgroups. Vulnerable populations— whether Southern blacks in the 1976 survey or individuals with chronic illness in the 1986 survey—have always been a major focus of the Foundation's interest. It is thus disturbing to find that access for vulnerable subpopulations may be deteriorating. In our early analyses of the 1994 data, we are giving particular attention to the uninsured—not focusing on the numbers of people without insurance but on their use of health care services. Less emphasis is being placed on overall trends in the use of services and more on the differentials across population subgroups. Although declining physician visits might indicate that care is being managed more efficiently, what does it mean if visits are declining at different rates for those with and without insurance coverage? While analyses are still under way, preliminary results confirm our suspicions that access for the most vulnerable groups in our country has declined. Despite expansions in Medicaid eligibility at both the federal and state levels, there are those who are still excluded from our health care system. Although the safety net may be larger, it is farther from the ground and the fall is potentially more threatening. Studies of access to care must focus greater attention on holes that have appeared in the safety net, targeting specific vulnerable subgroups of the population for further study and exploring the policy solutions to problems of access. The 1994 access survey reflects our belief, as well as the Foundation's, that providing policy makers with appropriate and reliable information increases the likelihood that effective programs will be designed and implemented.

COORDINATING WITH OTHER SURVEY EFFORTS

One of the secondary benefits of the 1994 design was increasing dialogue between the public and private sectors about the responsibilities of foundations and the federal government in monitoring changes in access to care. Since the 1994 access survey was conducted by a federal agency, by law the project was coordinated with other federal data-collection activities. We have learned the importance of ongoing and close collaboration between The Robert Wood Johnson Foundation and the federal government, even if the Foundation's future access surveys are not directly linked to those conducted by the government. Although the federal government does not sponsor any health care surveys whose *primary* objective is to study access, there are a number of federal surveys that do allow analysis of access issues. These include the National Health Interview Survey, the Medicare Current Beneficiary Survey, and the Medical Expenditure Panel Survey (which will be conducted annually and replace the National Medical Expenditure Survey). The resources of private foundations such as The Robert Wood Johnson Foundation should augment rather than duplicate such efforts.

Future access surveys should also be designed with awareness of other Foundation-supported activities intended to measure trends in access to care, such as those of the Center for Studying Health System Change. The Center's first major activity is the design and implementation of the Community Tracking Study, a longitudinal study designed to measure the effects of various health systems on a number of outcomes, including those related to access.

The Community Tracking Study, as well as federal surveys, will follow the access-to-care experiences of the nation overall, as well as in twelve communities across the country. These surveys, however, are of limited value in analyzing the specific access barriers experienced by some of the nation's most vulnerable groups. Still, they can help the Foundation understand *which* groups are experiencing problems getting care, even though there may be too few surveyed persons in each group to permit more detailed analysis on *why* they are having problems or on the health-related outcomes that result.

Future access surveys can better inform policy makers if they carefully target those groups of people who continue to have trouble obtaining adequate health care. The tracking mechanisms already in place can be used to help the Foundation identify which groups need to be targeted at any given time. Because of the long delays required in procurement and approvals, the federal government is poorly suited to sponsor these types of small, targeted efforts; in contrast, the Foundation is in a unique position to develop quickly surveys focused on the identified populations.

Endnotes

1. D. Rogers and L. Aiken, "Foreword," in L. A. Aday, R. Andersen, and G. V. Fleming, *Health Care in the U.S.: Equitable for Whom?* (Beverly Hills: Sage Publications, 1980), p. 17.

2. Much of the chronicle of events is derived from J. D. Kasper and M. L. Berk, "Sociological Gains and Losses: The Case of the National Health Care Use and Expenditure Surveys," *American Sociologist* 19(3) (Fall 1988), 232–242.

3. L. A. Aday, G. V. Fleming, and R. Andersen, *Access to Medical Care in the U.S.: Who Has It, Who Doesn't* (Chicago: University of Chicago, Center for Health Administration Studies, 1984), p. vii.

4. Aday, Fleming, and Andersen (1984), p. 110.

5. H. E. Freeman, R. J. Blendon, L. H. Aiken, S. Sudman, C. F. Mullinix, and C. R. Corey, "Americans Report on Their Access to Health Care," *Health Affairs* (Spring 1987), 6–18.

6. Robert Wood Johnson Foundation, *Special Report: Updated Report on Access to Health Care for the American People* (Princeton, N.J.: author, 1983).

7. M. L. Berk, "Should We Rely On Polls?" *Health Affairs* (Spring I 1994), 299–300.

8. H. E. Freeman and M. F. Shapiro, "A Contemporary Perspective on Access to Health Care," unpublished manuscript (1992).

9. A. C. Monheit, "Underinsured Americans: A Review," *Annual Review of Public Health* 15 (1994), 461–485.

10. M. L. Berk, C. L. Schur, and J. C. Cantor, "Ability to Obtain Health Care: Recent Estimates from the Robert Wood Johnson Foundation National Access to Care Survey," *Health Affairs* (Fall 1995), 139–146; quote from p. 139.

CHAPTER FOUR

~~ Expertise Meets Politics
Efforts to Work with States

Beth A. Stevens
Lawrence D. Brown

Editors' Introduction

Over the past twenty years, state governments have emerged as critical players in health care. They have an important regulatory role and, as payers for medical care under Medicaid and other programs offering services for needy people, can affect the structure of the delivery system.

As states develop health policies, foundations can assist by providing resources for technical assistance, research, and analysis, and demonstration of new ideas. Foundations can also bring together individuals interested in state health policy to share ideas and experiences. The Robert Wood Johnson Foundation has supported more than fifteen national programs to help states improve health policy, health financing, and the delivery of health care services.

Beth Stevens, a senior program officer at The Robert Wood Johnson Foundation, has managed evaluations of some of the key state programs supported by the Foundation. Lawrence Brown is a political scientist and professor of public health at Columbia University. He has followed and evaluated the Foundation's state policy activities for some time. In this chapter, they explore the question of what effect the Foundation's investments have had on health policy at the state level. It is a difficult question to answer, given complex state political environments and the indirect roles—such as improving information and understanding of options—that foundations play. The authors describe various Foundation-supported programs, examine the problems of working on health care improvement at the state level, and offer suggestions for future approaches to state health policy development. At its core, however, Chapter Four is a case study of how the State Initiatives in Health Policy Program, which attempted to assist states in insurance and financing reform, unfolded in the periods just before and after the efforts at national health care reform during the first Clinton administration.

Since the failure of health reform, programs with states have come under attack by people who assert that foundations are imposing their own agendas and are controlling, rather than aiding, state governments. We believe these assertions are wrong, but they underscore the points made by Stevens and Brown that the process of policy development is highly political and that foundations can play only limited roles. Moreover, even in these limited roles, foundations are subject to attack.

Health reform comes hard in the United States because the policy issues on which it turns are complex and controversial. Increasing access and containing costs are policies that arouse conflicts over concepts of equity versus efficiency, social justice versus autonomy, and the polity versus the market. Less obvious, and less noticed, however, is the fact that health reform also triggers disagreements about *institutions,* especially about *which* level of government should settle policy conflicts. At times, policy science and public sensibilities favor a powerful national role; at other times, states inspire greater confidence. Those who tread federalist minefields in hopes of advancing health policy debates aim at moving targets: the national government, the fifty states, some subset of the states, or some combination of central and subnational jurisdictions. In analyzing success in health policy, the "what" and the "who" generally intertwine, creating complications above and beyond the substantive issues.

The ever-shifting dynamic of federal versus state reform is an unsettling fact of life for all actors intent on reforming the health care system. Philanthropic foundations, whose mission to improve health care draws them into working with federal, state, and private-sector policy makers, have constantly been forced to place bets on which level of government is the most promising venue for change at any particular time. Should a foundation work alongside the federal government in efforts to expand health care to underserved areas, for example, or should it rely on state government enthusiasm for such efforts?

The Robert Wood Johnson Foundation has often worked with government at each level in pursuit of its mission to improve the health and health care of the American people. Its programs range from research funded jointly with the federal government to assess the feasibility of measuring the quality of home health care to programs that give states funds to try insurance reforms. Some of these have borne fruit, with the adoption of innovations and further refinement of policies; others yield few tangible products but may generate useful knowledge about why options do not work. Unfortunately, there has been little careful exploration of the intriguing questions these projects raise: When should a foundation work with governments to further its goals? How does it decide which governments to work with? What lessons emerge from Foundation-government relations?

The two-and-a-half-decade history of Foundation interaction with national and state governments is long and complex. No one paper can fully explain the origins and outcomes of such interplay between philanthropy and government or delineate its myriad patterns. Therefore, this chapter takes on part of this complex task by limiting its focus to The Robert Wood Johnson Foundation's involvement with *state* governments. Are there any patterns that can be drawn from Foundation and state government efforts to tell us when, where, and how philanthropic activities can most effectively contribute to improvements in health care and health? Are there any lessons to tell us about the limits philanthropies face in their efforts to improve the public good?

WORKING WITH STATE GOVERNMENTS

American culture and politics have long entrusted many important functions to the states, both to manage better government activities in a large nation and to balance the power of the central government. In health care, the states license physicians, nurses, hospitals, and health plans; run the Medicaid program; regulate capital spending (if they choose); and sponsor and subsidize various public health activities, such as immunizations and control of contagious diseases. The states often exceed the call of such duties by launching ambitious policy experiments to expand insurance coverage and control costs. Before President Bill Clinton offered his national plan in 1993, an impressive number of states—Hawaii, Washington, Massachusetts, Oregon, Minnesota, Vermont, Florida, and others—had made significant steps toward expanding coverage.

Issuing licenses and running public health programs logically fall to state governments, which after all are responsible for managing or monitoring local conditions. And health care, at least until recently, has been predominantly local, with most Americans receiving their care from community-based hospitals and physicians in private practice. But pursuing ambitious experiments in financing health care is a less obvious task for state governments to undertake. Such reforms often tread on national-level issues and dynamics; they can involve reallocation of federal funds and regulation of interstate commerce. So why do states take on these issues? What are the advantages of pursuing health care reform at the state level rather than the federal?

One reason is that states can test reform strategies and discover the advantages and limitations on a smaller scale. States can study each other's handiwork and emulate strategies if and as they choose. If innovations in one or more states look especially promising, they might even find their way into national policy—policy built on subnational learning instead of (or as well as) sophisticated theorizing. Second, states can tailor programs to their own conditions. The vagaries of disease, equity in access, medical science, the laws of supply and demand, and other staples of health reform may not respect state boundaries, but as the melodrama of 1992–1994 shows, differences among and within the fifty states vastly complicate the task of forming a consensus on national health policies. Liberals and conservatives differ as to how far variations among states should be respected in public policy, but all recognize that a diverse society requires variations on themes as well as common, integrative leitmotifs that pull the country together. Thus, reforms based on states can more closely fit the particular prevailing circumstances of geography, ethnic predominance, economic infrastructure, and political culture.

A third virtue of state control over health reforms is the states' superior "closeness to the people." The recent federal reform proposal collapsed in part because its creators did not adequately gauge the public's fear that Washington would impose alien arrangements on local institutions. State governments often appear to be more in tune with grass-roots values than is distant Washington. Leaving health reform to the states may or may not make it easier to resolve the major conflicts of value and interest on which health politics turn, but closeness to the public may at least make state endeavors less threatening than a full-tilt national push.

Although such arguments can be adduced to promote states as leaders in health reform, a host of practicalities complicates that ambitious mission. Fifty state systems compete with one another for such economic advantages as business investment, strong tax bases, and job growth. These economic goals are in tension with the increased fiscal extractions (higher taxes and employer mandates) and sizable redistributive measures that major health reforms demand. States that get too ambitious in reforming health care risk losing ground to competitor states. Leadership in health care reform can be a costly eccentricity.

Another practicality that constrains state innovation is federal policy. Medicare and Medicaid rules limit the power of the states to reroute roughly half the dollars in the system, and provisions of the

Employee Retirement and Income Security Act (ERISA) preclude state regulation of employer health plans. But even if these encumbrances were set aside, state health reform efforts, like their national counterparts, might still founder on the facts of political life. Change (let alone "fundamental" change) in health affairs is intrinsically contentious, and downsizing these battles from Washington to the states is no panacea for settling them. In fact, the states' closeness to the people may merely intensify the conflicts or smother them. Thus, state government assumption of the role of reformer is fraught with difficulties. Sometimes states can generate meaningful reforms, and sometimes they cannot.

FOUNDATION PROGRAMS: ENDS AND MEANS

In assessing the prospects for working with states to improve health and health care, foundations face the same perplexing package of advantages and disadvantages as do other agents for change. The key question is, what are the conditions that promote effective state-oriented foundation programs? Three factors are central to a foundation's ability to answer this question: the goals it wants to achieve, the strategies it uses to pursue them, and the fit between them.

GOALS

Since 1991, the Foundation has tried to improve health and health care by aiming at three concrete goals: to ensure that Americans of all ages have access to affordable basic health care, to improve the way services are organized and provided to people with chronic health conditions, and to promote health and prevent disease by reducing the harm caused by substance abuse. The Foundation has sponsored programs that work with state governments in pursuit of each of these goals.

To improve access to care, the Foundation has launched programs to expand insurance coverage for the uninsured. In the program State Initiatives in Health Care Reform, the Foundation helped states plan and develop significant innovations in financing, including insurance markets and Medicaid. The Health Care for the Uninsured Program supported the development and implementation of state and local initiatives to ensure the availability of health care services for those who lack insurance. It funded projects that designed and marketed insurance products, as well as those that sought to reduce various barriers (such as lack of information) that prevented markets from functioning effectively. The Making the Grade program encourages state governments to finance health services for school-age children by funding school-based clinics. States in this program try to forge links between clinics and new financing initiatives by reorganizing state and local funding policies. The Healthy Kids Program is an effort to assist selected states in design and development of insurance for school children. It uses Foundation funds to provide expert assistance to states so they can test and market these new products. Finally, the Foundation funded the Medicaid Managed Care Program, which works with state governments to maintain and improve access for vulnerable populations now covered under Medicaid managed care. Its intent is to build capacity among state governments, consumers, providers, and managed care plans to make managed care work for Medicaid enrollees.

Another set of programs helps state governments improve services for chronically ill people. The Program to Promote Long-Term Care Insurance for the Elderly stimulated public/private state-level partnerships to develop insurance covering long-term care services. The Foundation followed that program with State Initiatives in Long-Term Care, which offers funds to update long-term care financing and delivery systems. These might include integration of acute and long-term care, increased choice among financing options, and expanded coverage of long-term care services under Medicaid. Recently, the Foundation created the Medicare/Medicaid Integration Program to sponsor a ten-state demonstration of the dual-eligibility managed care model. This model integrates long-term and acute care services for elderly patients under combined Medicaid and Medicare capitated payments. The Foundation also funds work to improve the health care provided to other types of chronically ill Americans. In a project cosponsored with the Pew Charitable Trusts, it has funded experts from the Medicaid Working Group to provide technical assistance to states trying to integrate chronically ill and disabled people into Medicaid managed care systems. Finally, there is the Mental Health Services Program for Youth, which works to improve services for children with serious mental illness by supporting state agency consortia to change the financing, organization, and delivery of services.

In recent years, the Foundation has developed state-oriented programs to help reduce the harmful effects of substance abuse. Two major programs—Smokeless States and Reducing Underage Drinking Through Coalitions—fall into this category. The former provides money to strengthen state-level tobacco prevention and control initiatives aimed at children. The latter supports statewide coalitions of community organizations that publicize the benefits of reducing underage drinking and seek to implement plans to reach that goal.

In addition to pursuing its three specific goals, the Foundation works with states to reduce the costs of health care by focusing on the cost of programs that the states, rather than the federal government, fund. The Workers' Compensation Health Initiative funds demonstrations and evaluations of system reforms, such as inclusion of workers' compensation medical care in managed care systems and development of so-called "twenty-four-hour coverage" that integrates workers' compensation with medical and/or disability insurance.

Cutting across all substantive goals are the Information for State Health Policy program and the Intergovernmental Health Policy Project at the National Conference of State Legislators, both of which seek to build and increase the general policy-making capacity of state governments. The former gives funds to state governments enabling them to improve their ability to collect and report data on the health and health care of their citizens, while the latter enables the conference to organize seminars and prepare educational materials about health policy issues for state legislators.

STRATEGIES

Four basic strategies constitute the fundamental philanthropic approaches to helping state governments improve their policies affecting health and health care. Each one aims to overcome a key obstacle to effective policy development.

The first philanthropic approach is providing funds to convene parties whose formal agreement or informal influence is essential to solving the health care problems in question. "Bringing the parties together" is a necessary condition of action; such activities can range from informal working groups to formal, multiyear state commissions. The Mental Health Services Program for Youth, for example, promoted such "convening" by sponsoring meetings of officials of disparate, competitive state agencies and advocacy groups so that common procedures and funding could be negotiated. This was an integral part of the program's work to break down categorical barriers to comprehensive services for young people.

The second technique is building the capacity of state government officials to analyze problems and craft solutions. State government officials have complex duties in dozens of policy arenas. Securing the full-time services of talented staff people who focus on limited issues increases the likelihood that coherent and practical health reform plans will emerge and that the proposals will be well-represented, even championed, by the governor's office or legislative leaders. The Program to Promote Long-Term Care Insurance, for example, provided funds so that state officials could devote their time to the task of designing and promoting this new form of insurance—a process that required coordination among underwriters, demographers, marketing experts, agencies for the aging, and claims processors.

The third approach is providing technical assistance to state officials to enhance their ability to address complicated policy issues. Here the Foundation seeks to eliminate factual or analytic roadblocks to both policy development and political consensus. If, for example, the governor's office or key legislators want to clarify an issue, they may request funding of a special study or the services of expert consultants. The Foundation gave state grantees funds to hire experts to construct state expenditure accounts in the State Initiatives in Health Care Reform Program and paid for actuarial analyses that underlie state-sponsored insurance programs in the Healthy Kids and Partnerships in Long-Term Care Insurance programs.

The fourth and final approach is promoting interchange among reformers and policy makers in different states. By holding annual meetings for all its grantees in state-oriented programs, funding publication of newsletters and technical documents, and centralizing administration of its programs in national program offices headed by experts, the Foundation facilitates diffusion of ideas from one state to another. The networks of state reformers have the potential to provide mutual support, share possible solutions to common problems, and create a cadre of states pressing for the resolution of particular health problems. This technique has been particularly prominent in the Mental Health Services Program for Youth and Smokeless States programs.

CASE STUDY: THE STATE INITIATIVES PROGRAM

All these programs differ widely, not only in their policy targets and their strategies for creating social change but also in their ambition. Some are aimed at a relatively narrow target, such as helping states design health insurance products for children; others work for broader changes, such as restructured long-term care financing. Similarly, some programs use a few of the philanthropic tools, while others use a mixture of all four. One of the most ambitious programs the Foundation has developed over the past twenty years is State Initiatives in Health Care Reform. The program offers the opportunity to analyze a program that sets complex goals and uses most of the strategies that foundations have available: convening, technical assistance, staff support, and communications among states. The program shows how generic philanthropic ends and means can help improve health care—as well as how they can be twisted into unexpected outcomes by refractory state political dynamics. It offers an exceptionally instructive case study of the ups and downs of Foundation efforts to encourage changes in health policy.

The State Initiatives in Health Care Reform Program was authorized in 1991, before Bill Clinton was elected and made national health care reform a national preoccupation. In 1991, the prospects for achieving access to health care for all Americans (one of the Foundation's major goals) were fairly dim. The Bush Administration, like the Reagan Administration before it, proposed only limited changes in the way most Americans received insurance coverage for their health care. If access were to be expanded, the Foundation reckoned, it was more likely to come through state-level action. Twenty-eight states had already convened commissions to study proposed reforms in health care financing; a smaller number had received waivers from the federal government to expand their Medicaid programs. In many states, governors and legislators were talking up reforms and debating authorizing legislation. The political will to make major reforms in health care financing appeared to be in place or en route. These considerations moved the Foundation to authorize up to $25.5 million for awards to as many as fifteen state governments to advance the development of significant reforms in health care financing on the state level. (The program was subsequently reauthorized on two occasions. In 1993, the original program, which had ultimately funded twelve states, was expanded to eight more. In 1996, the Foundation decided to maintain its support of state-level reform by providing fifteen states—both recipients and new applicants—with $7.5 million more in grants, to run until the year 2001.)

The explicit goal of the program has been to help states plan and develop insurance market and Medicaid reforms that expand health insurance coverage for the uninsured while slowing the rise in health care costs. Grantees have examined a variety of options, ranging from New Mexico's exploration of universal health insurance coverage through a state-sponsored program to Oregon's employer mandate (enacted and then deferred) and Florida's innovative insurance purchasing pools.

The Foundation deliberately used most of the tools at its disposal. Recognizing that few states had the personnel and financial resources needed to develop and implement health care financing reform, it authorized funds for states to hire or reassign employees who would work on the issue.

Internal capacity is only part of the story, however. Without expertise to guide them, states might stall or resort to unworkable quick fixes. The Foundation's program designers therefore secured technical expertise from a central pool of nationally recognized research organizations. The Urban Institute was funded to help states track trends in eligibility and coverage under state programs and to simulate the effects of policy changes on the uninsured and Medicaid populations. The Rand Corporation helped states analyze the consequences of specific policy options for the state budget, total spending on health, and different sectors of the health care market. The National Governor's Association worked with states to understand policy options for, and barriers to, health financing reform. It, too, produced reports, such as an analysis of the impact of ERISA on state options, and also provided a forum for states to share and discuss policy issues.

The staff time and the technical assistance were devoted to helping states one-by-one. Although such help is obviously important, reforms seldom occur in isolation. Reformers benefit by comparing notes on options that look promising or possibilities that became dead ends. The Foundation therefore funded the Alpha Center so that states could help one another create a wave of reform. Alpha convened conferences on technical and strategic issues; issued newsletters, reports, and other documents; and publicized efforts of individual grantees to a wider audience.

THE RESULTS OF FOUNDATION ACTIVITIES

Although no state has yet entered the promised land of affordable universal coverage, the State Initiatives program has helped states in several ways to map, and sometimes to navigate, the twisting road toward it.

The first philanthropic strategy—providing funds to convene stake-holders in health reform—was embraced by most state grantees. Many, including Vermont, Montana, and West Virginia, used Foundation funds to establish special commissions or task forces charged with developing and discussing options for financing care. To be sure, these commissions did not lead to wholesale system reform, but Foundation-funded task forces put such changes high on the agendas of many key public and private stakeholders. Would these discussions have taken place without philanthropic funds? Financing reform was pursued by states outside the program, such as Hawaii, Tennessee, and Massachusetts; and some state grantees had initiated substantial changes in health financing policy before the program began (Minnesota, Washington, Florida, and Oregon, to name the most prominent). One can never control completely for the many intersecting variables that shape innovations and therefore cannot isolate Foundation influence more than impressionistically, but in some grantee states the issue of coverage for the uninsured probably gained more prominence than if the program had not existed.

The second Foundation strategy—providing funds for states to hire staff that would be devoted to the development of policy options—sustained a concentrated and penetrating exploration of promising, albeit complicated, ideas. In Colorado, a five-person policy office designed state-licensed purchasing pools and developed a way to adjust Medicaid payments for risk. New York staff analyzed whether it would make sense to extend the states' all-payer regulations to individual physicians (evidently not) and whether to expand community rating to insured groups larger than fifty. Similar analyses proceeded in other states, which gained a surer grasp of the pros and cons of policy proposals.

Program-funded technical assistance to state grantees reinforced the internal abilities enhanced by the other strategies. The Urban Institute produced reports such as the "State Level Data Book" and "The Distributional Effects of Employer Mandates." These offered information and analyses available nowhere else because they used statistical models that few could match. Researchers from the Rand Corporation designed and analyzed a survey of employers and households in the ten original program states in order to provide much needed state-based estimates of insurance benefits and coverage, and thus a more accurate picture of the state's uninsured population. Rand experts also helped states develop State Health Expenditure Accounts, which let states see where their health care dollars went. The Urban

Institute's simulation model, "Trim 2," let states test by how much various policy options increased coverage for uninsured populations. Both the Urban Institute and the Rand researchers worked as consultants to the states as well, for example by organizing educational retreats for state legislators who were eager to explore the technical aspects of different policy options. The Alpha Center encouraged new policy options by holding conferences on such topics as innovative state/Medicaid purchasing strategies; monitoring risk-bearing entities; and the implications of the Health Insurance Portability and Accountability Act of 1996 (the "Kassebaum-Kennedy" legislation). Alpha's reports on issues such as the utility of subsidies to low-income individuals for the purchase of insurance and the lessons of state efforts to develop standardized benefits packages helped build a knowledge base across the states.

Finally, the program advanced communication of ideas and experiences among state grantees and from the states as a group to national deliberations. Conferences, working groups, and technical documents built a sense of community among state reformers. Minnesota representatives shared its incremental approaches to expanded coverage with numerous states; New York explained its electronic claims clearinghouses to Maryland; North Dakota learned from Vermont how to collect data on health expenditures; and Nebraska looked to Iowa for ideas about the design of private insurance purchasing cooperatives. Such sharing helped states avoid policy pitfalls and dead ends and enhanced their understanding of the strategies and stakes of innovation. State leaders and other policy experts now know more about how to subsidize the working poor to help them buy insurance without also encouraging employers to cut their own contributions to workers' coverage in hope of getting a subsidy. States are learning how to pool insurance purchasers to gain economies of scale, as well as market leverage, as Florida, Minnesota, Colorado, and Iowa have done. These insights are significant contributions to future policy debates.

NECESSARY BUT NOT SUFFICIENT: LIMITS OF FOUNDATION SUPPORT

The improvements in policy design and deliberation that foundation strategies produce are noteworthy contributions, but they fall short of achieving broad-ranging (and often even narrow-gauged) reform. No foundation program, including The Robert Wood Johnson Foundation's State Initiatives, has made a major dent in the problems of the uninsured in the states. By 1997, after almost a decade of intermittent but often intense deliberations, no state had achieved universal coverage, none (save Hawaii) had implemented an employer mandate, none had comprehensively reformed its health care system, and most watched the number of uninsured rise steadily despite relatively good economic times. These realities are not so much a verdict of failure, however, as a spotlight on our central point: foundation programs such as State Initiatives may be necessary (or, at any rate, highly useful) to help states down the road to reform, but they are far from sufficient. In a democracy, foundations cannot and should not be expected to engineer reform because conflicts of values and interests in the states themselves demand, and deserve, free play. To an account of goals and strategies, then, one should add the third piece of the policy puzzle, namely, the political characteristics of the states that shape and transform the work of foundations.

Whether foundation programs, such as State Initiatives, end up "working" or not depends largely on the funder's sagacity in reading the capacity and political personality of state applicants. Unfortunately, foundation appraisers usually have little pertinent information on which to rely. A large research literature maps correlates of state liberalism and conservatism in social policy, but these studies have many conceptual and methodological limits and, in any case, shed little light on the disparate factors that might predict the capacity of states to tackle particular reforms. Moreover, states that seem to be quite similar on objective measures (such as the level of economic development) can vary dramatically in policy behavior. Because innovation is, by definition, a significant departure from past practice, it is anyone's guess what information would be needed by funders to predict the probability that innovations will occur and succeed. Because off-the-shelf intimations of state capacity are few and poor, foundations must resort to rough-and-ready indicators such as the stature and commitment of key players representing the state in its quest for money, the state's reputation within policy networks for competence, track records in previous programs, the prospects for public and private-sector collaboration, and the copiousness and cogency of the documents submitted. Meanwhile, prediction becomes all the more imponderable because foundations are typically hoping to nudge states to "higher" levels of policy consciousness, eventually crowned by consensus on major reform.

Even if states were equally positioned for reform, the strategies that philanthropies use have distinct limitations. Convening the parties interested in financing reform, although necessary to begin moving toward consensus, is rarely without risk. One never knows in advance where such deliberations will lead. Sometimes dialogue breeds trust and a sense of collective will, but sometimes it reminds participants why they dodged each other in the past and why they can at best agree to disagree. Sometimes it encourages solutions with a lowest common denominator, whose virtue is that they threaten no one at the table. Making agreements stick, moreover, is complicated by turnover in key positions. Governors and legislators, such as those in Washington and Kentucky, who set and pushed the reform agenda are not around to help guide it into law or, alternatively, to help implement laws they passed. Elected state leaders regularly lose office or influence by means of retirement, electoral defeat, shifts from majority to minority party, and other misfortunes that remove them from the reform game. Frequently, reforming states end up entrusting complex proposals and fledgling laws to the ministrations of public and private leaders who may know little (and care less) about how they emerged and what they meant, and who may doubt their wisdom or even oppose them outright. Shifts in political fortunes in Massachusetts in the late 1980s, and Florida in 1994, for example, display this type of change in painful detail. A foundation has trouble encouraging the convening of stakeholders and thus beginning the process of reform when those who ought to be convened and the issues they need to discuss keep changing.

Technical assistance, the most favored tool of foundations because it is easily produced, runs into contradictions. Because reform is a significant departure from past practice, it is difficult to guess what type of information will be needed to create solutions to complicated and value-laden problems. Moreover, particular state conditions demand particularized solutions, for which the standardized national-level technical assistance that foundations provide might be inappropriate. Finally, immersion in "the data" can multiply and diffuse issues and options, instead of narrowing or focusing them. In 1993, for example, the Foundation-funded project in Minnesota developed higher estimates of the number of uninsured than the state had been using. This created some disarray in the state political establishment and disrupted progress toward a political solution.

In the end, technical assistance cannot completely resolve the complex debates over health reform because it runs into political reality.

Ultimately, the health reform plans devised by the best and the brightest experts must pass tests of political acceptability. Foundation aid that expands data and analyses that make the development of proposals easier (and doubtless better) may also deflect attention from political realities. Some otherwise excellent plans (in the technical sense) devised by state technocrats affronted the sensibilities of an uncomprehending public and of an all-too-comprehending phalanx of interest groups whose political interests conflicted with the plans. In places like Vermont, Colorado, and Kentucky, such conflict provoked a backlash that caused the downfall of the "technically superior" plan. It is relatively easy for foundations to help set agendas; it is beyond their mandate to bring reform to legislative life.

Convening, providing technical expertise, offering state staff the time and the resources to pursue reform, and even the camaraderie of membership in a program with other states working toward the same purposes can enhance political deliberations but cannot settle political disagreement. Expanding health coverage is a complicated exercise that requires cooperation from purchasers (public, private, individual), beneficiaries (who may or may not be purchasers and who may contribute to the costs of "reform" in the coin of premiums, copayments, forgone wages, and otherwise), subsidy sources, providers (physicians, hospitals, nursing homes), and of course insurance firms, too. These players, caught in the dynamics of managed care and consolidation even as foundation programs unfold, are not always captains of their fate and may not be reliable program partners. Moreover, such projects can involve a number of state agencies—departments of health, insurance, social services, aging—whose preferences may differ from those of private-sector stakeholders (and of other public agencies). Resolution of conflicts is more often a matter of political compromise and difference splitting than of analytical enlightenment. Politics, however messy, is the sole practical means of resolving the conflict among values and interests.

Foundations and those who evaluate their work should recognize that discussion, better staffing, technical aid, and diffusion of knowledge can tidy up the messiness of health politics only so far. Some conflicts are, so to speak, "hardwired" into complex policy problems by the very nature of decision making in a democratic society. One enduring complication is the range of stakeholders in state health policy and their divergent interests. When seeking to promote subnational change, foundations are not simply dealing with a coherent, unitary entity called "the state"; rather, they must work with many independent organizations, public and private. Insurance reform, for example, may engage the departments of insurance and health as well as the governor and staff and various legislators and committees. How these public bodies behave will also partly reflect preferences of private actors: the insurance industry, managed care organizations, provider associations, employer groups. Lucky is the foundation program that minimizes the number of stakeholders and thus shortens the chain of potentially contentious political clearances. For instance, Medicaid reforms for the disabled do not much implicate employers and insurers, and innovations in long-term care coverage have little direct impact on providers (other than nursing homes). Generally, however, reform requires the support (or at least the acquiescence) of numerous public agencies and private groups who want to know why and how it is in their interests to cooperate. Mandating or convincing them to participate, however, lies beyond the foundation's reach.

A second persistent fact of political life is the intensity of the players' preferences and of conflicts among them. If health policy problems admitted straightforward moral or empirical answers, they would presumably have been resolved long ago. Reform comes hard because health affairs evoke deep disagreement about "the facts," their moral meaning, and their implications for stakeholders.

These intrinsic tensions, however, limit the efficacy of foundations, for whom politics must remain a spectator sport. Innovative insurance offerings, perhaps accompanied by public subsidies, look like a plausible strategy for enticing small business firms to start buying health insurance for their workers—or so a foundation may suppose. When such voluntary efforts fail, however, a foundation cannot overcome business opposition to an employer mandate. Foundation-funded programs only flourish with the invention of win-win designs that benefit all sides. Foundations cannot mandate change in the face of opposition. Win-win programs are not impossible—public-private partnerships in long-term care insurance seem to fill the bill, though critics question whether consumers who pay hefty annual premiums are true winners—but they seldom come easily.

WHAT IS TO BE DONE?

Foundations are condemned to falter in pursuit of health reform because their goals are high, the means available to them are limited, and health reform combines complicated policy problems with acute political conflicts. These constraints on activism mean that The Robert Wood Johnson Foundation's state-based programs must often make do with leading to the waters of policy wisdom horses it cannot compel to drink.

This is not to say, however, that the Foundation's efforts to improve state health policy are ineffective or inefficient. The interposition of foundation and other "third force" institutions between the public and private sectors carries its frustrations but also unique opportunities for innovation. Insulated from both long chains of clearance and electoral sensibilities in government, and from demands for a quick, high return from shareholders of corporations, a foundation can conceive and field innovations limited only by its imagination, funds, and sense of what is workable and in keeping with its mission. It is not to be expected that such gambits will "work" well—or at all—every time, everywhere. Talking and analyzing may not much stir the blood of those who would have the states adopt affordable universal coverage immediately, but interventions that bridge the stages of the stammering social conversation that is health reform are no small feat, especially given the glacial progress of consensus in the states.

The true strategic challenge for a foundation is to avoid either ignoring or indulging the realities of health politics in the states, and instead to "read" these fifty polities for signs indicating how best to advance and accelerate reform. For example, programs tend to run more smoothly and achieve better outcomes when they do not implicate the interests of many groups, when group conflicts over ends or means are not deep and intense, and when the technology of problem solving is relatively straightforward. The Foundation's Program to Promote Long-Term Care Insurance for the Elderly seems to meet these criteria. The key players are departments of health (and/or insurance) and the insurance industry. Obligations and costs can be divided in ways that make economic sense for budget makers, Medicaid programs, insurers, consumers, and nursing homes. Writing and selling such insurance policies (even with appropriate protections for consumers) is not rocket science. Programs to expand coverage for the uninsured, by contrast, have needed support from employers, workers, providers, insurers, and public subsidy sources. None of these groups warmed to the effort, and most saw at least as many costs as benefits to themselves in participating. Writing coverage that was both attractive and affordable was complex indeed.

The Robert Wood Johnson Foundation may want to retain ambitious reform goals, but it may also seek means to assess risks more precisely in advance and to target interventions to more particular political conditions. Doing so requires, first, a systematic reading of the political complexion of the states (are they at the stage of talking, analyzing, or legislating, and how likely are they to master that stage and move successfully to the next?) and second, close contemplation of the main players in the reform "game," in terms of the depth of conflicts among their values and interests and the prospects that they might endorse an intervention that they can implement effectively. Program strategies must then be designed to fit the many realities of different states.

We have come full circle. Health reform comes hard in the United States because the issues are complex and controversial. Both expertise—to devise feasible solutions—and politics—to achieve consensus on solutions—are necessary to achieve true change in state health policy. Foundations can initiate the process—setting the challenge, providing resources to explore the possible answers, and in general enhancing the quality of the debate. But foundations cannot settle that debate. In the final analysis, it is the states and politics that sort out the differing preferences and values that shape true health care reform.

CHAPTER FIVE

The Media and Change in Health Systems

Marc S. Kaplan
Mark A. Goldberg

Editors' Introduction

Since the Foundation emerged as a national philanthropy a quarter century ago, research has been one of its strategies for helping the nation (albeit indirectly) improve the health and health care of Americans. The logic of the investments in research presumes that more-reliable information can be the basis of more-informed public debates and decision making about health care.

However, the Foundation's interest in research has always been an applied one: it is funded to the extent that it advances—even if in the long run—the goals that are the cornerstones of the Foundation's grant making. However, for research to have an impact, it must be disseminated. Traditionally, research findings by grantees have been communicated through articles in peer-reviewed academic journals.

Although not deemphasizing the importance of peer-reviewed publications, in recent years the Foundation has recognized the importance of getting information to audiences other than academics and policy experts. Chapter Five describes one experience with an ambitious effort to communicate research findings to a wider audience. The Local

Media Education Project was a program to transmit to journalists the latest research on the changing health care system in their communities and to explain what it meant for their readers.

Even though the idea of getting findings to local journalists is easy to state, implementing it turned out to be time-consuming and difficult. The chapter takes the reader behind the scenes of one such effort, conducted by the authors, Marc S. Kaplan, a senior communications officer at The Robert Wood Johnson Foundation, and Mark A. Goldberg, a distinguished fellow at the Yale University School of Management and a senior fellow at the Carnegie Foundation for the Advancement of Teaching. It provides insights about how foundations can work to ensure that findings from their grant-supported research reach diverse audiences.

Health care in the United States has increasingly become managed care, and just about everybody is perplexed about the pace, the direction, and the implications of the change coursing through their local institutions and markets. Yet, despite their confusion, people must make decisions: patients about their selections among health care plans, providers, and courses of treatment; providers about their responsibilities as professionals in a shifting environment; employers about the extent and the types of health care insurance to buy or subsidize for employees; managers of health care organizations and insurers about their strategies for survival and success; and public officials about how to manage and adjust government health care programs in the midst of change.

Change seems to characterize health care everywhere: in large cities and small towns, in every region of the country. But that change is not uniform. Every local market is distinctive in its history, its set of health care institutions and players, its demographic and health profile, its culture, and its competitive dynamic. Much of what can be done to explain health care change, therefore, has to be done at a local level—in the idiosyncratic markets where people live and work and where each group must make decisions about care and its financing and delivery. That is why The Robert Wood Johnson Foundation funded the Local Media Education Project. This project had two components: briefings of print journalists in fourteen cities and briefings of broadcast journalists in four of those cities.

WHY BRIEF JOURNALISTS ABOUT HEALTH SYSTEMS CHANGE?

Our briefings proceeded from four premises. The first was a broad conception of the potential audience for health systems research. We believed that the results of some (though certainly not all) such research would interest not only analysts and public policy makers but also the consumers of health services, whose well-being and finances could be affected by changes under way in health systems, and a range of key actors in the private and nonprofit sectors.

The second premise was that journalists are themselves a crucial audience for the results of research about health system change, because they inform and help shape the understandings of other audiences. Journalists alert consumers to developments and potential developments that involve their interests. They also apprise key health care decision makers of developments in and outside their particular segments of the system. Key health care players pay close attention to the major newspapers in their communities, as sources of information about what other players are doing or planning to do and for insights into the perceptions and concerns of consumers.

A third basis for our briefings was that the Center for Studying Health System Change had generated a body of research that could be extraordinarily useful to journalists as they reported on changes in local health care markets. The Center, which is based in Washington, D.C., was established and funded by The Robert Wood Johnson Foundation to track and analyze health systems changes around the country. In its first phase of work, the Community Snapshots Project, the Center assembled brief profiles, or "snapshots," of developments in fifteen markets, selected to represent a range of regions, population sizes, and stages of development. Each market was covered by one of three teams of researchers, whether from the Alpha Center in Washington, D.C., the University of California at San Francisco, or the University of Washington. The teams conducted extensive local interviews and reviewed secondary materials. They prepared reports on the nature and sources of change in that market: the experiences, reactions, and strategies of major actors in that market, including providers, purchasers, insurers and health plans, public policy makers, and consumers; and the potential trajectory of the market.[1] On the basis of these snapshots, the Center and members of the three research teams also were able to develop cross-cutting analyses that identified and explored similarities and differences in the patterns observed across communities.[2]

In addition, the Foundation commissioned Louis Harris and Associates to undertake a broad survey of consumers, including a nationally representative sample of 605 respondents and separate representative samples of approximately 300 respondents in each of the fifteen markets studied. Consumers in both the national and market-specific surveys were asked three broad sets of questions: about their perceptions of trends in access to health care and its cost and quality; about their reactions to the growing influx and influence of managed care, and about their expectations and concerns for the future.[3]

Here, then, was a wealth of material that could help journalists refine their understanding of the changes taking place in their communities' health care markets, the interplay among sets of actors and interests, and the perceptions and reactions of consumers (their readers). What is more, because fifteen markets had been analyzed concurrently within a common framework, and because surveys had been conducted in those markets and nationally with a common instrument, we were able to draw comparisons across markets and, for the survey results, relate the response patterns in an individual community to those in the national sample.

The fourth predicate for this initiative was that the Center's work potentially had value to journalists over time as well as in the short term. The Center's findings—particularly the results of the market-specific surveys—were news, and we hoped that they would be covered as such. But we also hoped that our briefings about the site visit reports and the surveys would make a more lasting contribution—that they would help journalists place future news stories in context for their readers. Our effort was meant to educate, not only to disseminate. That is why, within The Robert Wood Johnson Foundation, it came to be known as the Local Media Education Project.

BRIEFINGS OF PRINT JOURNALISTS

In the spring of 1996, under the auspices of the Foundation, the two authors of this chapter visited fourteen markets out of the fifteen studied, in which health care providers, insurers, employers, public officials, and, not least, patients are living through a period of consolidation, competition, and dislocation. In our visits, we met with journalists who cover the transformation of those markets. We briefed newspaper reporters and editors on changes in their specific market, with information from research conducted under the auspices of the Center for Studying Health System Change.

We met with an average of four journalists at each of the newspapers we visited. At fourteen of the fifteen newspapers, our briefings were attended not only by reporters but also by editors. The presence of editors was significant because they decide a newspaper's priorities—what reporters are assigned to cover, what topics and stories find their way into print. At seven of the newspapers, we spoke with editorial writers, too.

Briefings were constructed from five sets of materials: (1) the site visit reports for the fifteen markets studied; (2) the results from the market-specific surveys and the national poll conducted by Louis Harris and Associates; (3) updated reports for each of the markets, typically written by one of the original analysts on the basis of follow-up interviews and a review of secondary materials; (4) newspaper articles, found in NEXIS searches, about health system changes in each market since the site visit reports were completed; and (5) the researchers' analysis of patterns and trends across markets. The meetings we had with editors and reporters were highly interactive and fluid. We invited journalists to jump in at any time with questions or observations, and they did.

We started each session by describing The Robert Wood Johnson Foundation and its work and, in turn, the Center for Studying Health System Change, its Community Snapshots Project, and its research program. Next, we summarized the broad patterns of change, causation, and strategies found across the fifteen communities. Distinctive features of the particular market under discussion were highlighted, framing, with themes and potential story lines, the market-specific details to follow. Journalists at virtually every newspaper we visited wanted to know what was special about their area's health care market—what set it apart from the others studied.

The next (and longest) portion of the briefing was a discussion of the major players, directions and drivers of change, and patterns of competition. We also listed emerging trends and potential developments in the market—trends and developments that might warrant future coverage. The final component of the presentation at each newspaper was an examination of the findings of the Harris survey in the local market and a comparison of them with findings in the national survey.

The participating journalists were knowledgeable and energetic. They asked all sorts of questions, about their markets, other markets, the workings of competition, and managed care. As busy as these journalists were, they stayed put for our briefings, each of which lasted an average of two hours. The Local Media Education Project led to a first wave of thirty articles or editorials in the fourteen markets we visited. Every newspaper ran at least one story about the research conducted by the center and its collaborators. Five newspapers ran front-page stories: the *Orange County Register* (California); the *Gainesville Sun*; the *Indianapolis Star*; the *Forum* in Fargo, North Dakota; and the *Des Moines Register*. Two papers put articles about the center's findings on page one of the metro or regional section, and three others on the front page of the business section.

As we had suspected they would, newspapers treated the results of surveys in their markets as news. But most of them did much more than simply report those results. They also put news from the surveys into context by comparing local response patterns to patterns in the national survey and by relating the findings of the survey to the characteristics of the local health care market, as described in the site visit reports and the briefings. Some of the newspapers also focused more directly on the findings of site visit reports about their markets and, drawing on the briefings, put those findings into context as well by comparing local markets to others that had been analyzed by the site visit teams. Four newspapers also published editorials that discussed the results and the implications of the site visits and surveys.

LESSONS LEARNED

Here are some of the lessons that we took away from our briefings that we hope others who are contemplating similar conversations with print journalists will find helpful.

Newness

In Fargo, Joe Dill, the editor of the *Forum,* asked us the single best question we heard in fifteen briefings: "In all of these materials about the Fargo health care market, what surprised you the most?" The question reminded us that surprise—or freshness, at least—is at the heart of most news. If findings are not new or surprising, maybe they are not, as viewed by journalists, newsworthy. They may, nevertheless, be important in framing news—that is, in providing context.

Meaning for Readers

At almost every session, journalists asked, in these words or a close approximation, "What does this"—a consolidation of hospitals, the proliferation of managed care, efforts to measure outcomes—"mean for our readers?" Journalists see themselves as surrogates and watchdogs for readers, looking out for their interests and asking questions on their behalf.

We offer three corollary observations. First, not all journalists at a newspaper define their readers identically. Thus, some business reporters asked us what particular phenomena might mean for employers, hospitals, or insurers; they were especially interested in overall cost trends and competitive impacts. Reporters for the main news or metro sections of newspapers tended to ask about effects on patients and consumers; they focused on quality of care and out-of-pocket costs. Second, if the answer to that central question, "What does this mean for our readers?" is "not much," chances are that that is a good estimate of how much coverage will be forthcoming. A health systems researcher who is contemplating an approach to journalists would be well advised to be ready with a more substantial and persuasive response; if none is possible regarding a particular research project, then perhaps that project, however worthy it may otherwise be, is just not prime material for journalists. Third, journalists know that the meaning of a development or a trend may be different for different readers. That is why they often ask, as many did in the briefings, "Who are the winners and the losers?"

The Distinctive Credibility of Researchers

Researchers, especially those affiliated with academic institutions or independent research organizations, have an advantage over others who seek to speak with journalists about health care: they are accorded a presumption not just of objectivity but of fairness—of freedom from, in particular, pecuniary motivations. Thus, one reporter told us that most of the people he hears from about health care issues "have an ax to grind" and "stand to make or lose a lot of money" in the local health care market; he exempted us from this characterization. Researchers may have a related advantage as well: the perception that they offer a fresh take. Here, for instance, is the opening sentence of a column by Eve Tahmincioglu, in the *News Journal,* about the site visit report for the Wilmington, Delaware, market: "It's always great to get the perspective of outsiders, especially when it comes to your community's health system."[4]

The Added Value of Context

Many of the journalists we met came to our briefings for news—the results of a survey of local consumers, the findings of a site visit report—but stayed for context. These briefings allowed them to step back from the day-to-day rush of new developments and to take in the big picture: not just the pieces but the dynamics of their local market; not just their local market but that market in comparison to others; not just current events but their causes, potential consequences, and possible trajectories. Many of the questions that journalists asked were about context and went beyond what they needed to know to write a story or two in the short run. Researchers who brief journalists should expect—and perhaps even encourage—questions that help reporters, editors, and editorial writers to refine and test their broader understandings.

The Usefulness of Face-to-Face Meetings

It takes time to meet with journalists, but our experience suggests that the extra effort pays dividends. A face-to-face conversation, at a scheduled time and away from the hubbub of a newsroom, allows for a more relaxed exploration of the issues raised by research and of the context of the work and findings. That exploration can contribute to a journalist's understanding and his or her ability over time to explain developments to readers—and it increases the chances of coverage, and better coverage, in the near future. The articles written after our briefing sessions about the findings of the Community Snapshots Project went farther in providing detail, linking survey results and site visit findings, and explaining context than they could or would have on the basis of a press release alone, or a press release supplemented by hurried telephone conversations with busy journalists on deadline.

BRIEFING BROADCAST JOURNALISTS

For several years now, the ratings for national news broadcasts have declined while the number of local television news viewers has grown steadily. An opportunity presented itself to launch a component of the Local Media Education Project targeting local television stations with information about the changing health care system in their communities. In conjunction with the Radio and Television News Directors Foundation, the Education Project held one-day seminars in Indianapolis, Houston, San Diego, and Miami. In each location, broadcast journalists were invited to a two-part program.

The first part consisted of an overview of the Snapshots report and Harris poll data, followed by panel discussions on recent or upcoming local health care developments. For the second part of the program, we went into the field, to health care settings where reporters could witness firsthand the consequences of their health system in flux. What was learned from discussions with seminar participants during the events, in questionnaires returned immediately after the seminars, and in lengthy telephone interviews six weeks later contributed to our understanding of how to present health care information to broadcast journalists, as distinguished from their newspaper counterparts.

Information in a newspaper story generally includes context, analysis, background, and various points of view. The three-dimensional character of this reporting is possible because of the longer lead time a print journalist usually has to research a story and the space allotted for its exposition. The constraints that television news imposes on the time a reporter has to research and report a story, and on the time allotted for it in an actual broadcast, are much different from those faced by print journalists. These constraints dictate not only how to present information to television reporters but also how to shape its substance so as to get it reported. News decisions for both television and newspapers are determined by whether an item directly or indirectly affects large numbers of people, and in what ways. The more salient (and, usually, the more disruptive), the more newsworthy. Ordinarily, television reporters can be approached only on the basis of news. For example, while the Snapshots report contained valuable information on the shifting dynamics of health care delivery in the markets of the television reporters, they regarded only the opinion polls as being able to cross the news threshold and make it onto a broadcast. In one market, which managed care had barely penetrated, it was not even possible to interest television reporters to attend a news briefing on the poll. The phenomenon of managed care simply hadn't reached a level where reporters considered it news.

But perhaps the most significant factor in how information gets treated on television news is time. Television reporters typically have at most three minutes to tell a story, and as a result nuance, complexity, and subtlety are sacrificed for generalization and oversimplification. This brief window allows comfortably for only two points of view on a single issue, contributing to the "he said/she said" phenomenon of television news. When panel discussions ventured into territory that is necessarily complex, such as a county moving its entire Medicaid population into managed care, evaluation forms came back complaining that the sessions were too technical, too detailed, too complicated.

A recurring criticism of the seminars was that the panel discussions did not sufficiently set the dynamics of the changing marketplace in dramatic relief. Television news, we were told, is about conflict. The diversity of opinions expressed in the panel discussions frustrated many broadcast reporters who wanted to be able to analyze developments in the health care system in terms of simple, clear-cut terms of winners and losers. Furthermore, we found that a single expert able to present two sides of an issue was of less interest to broadcast reporters than two individuals who were able to take opposite ends of the same issue. For example, journalists gave high marks to a panel discussion that contrasted one physician in favor of managed care with another highly critical of it.

Another great divide between print and television journalism lies in their respective abilities to use numbers to tell a story. Clearly, television is a medium driven by images to tell a story. Numbers in the form of charts and tables impede the narrative flow. When the Harris Poll results were reported on the news, for example, they took the form of a graph that was on and off the screen before viewers could absorb it. If numbers are to be depicted pictorially on television, they need to be presented with the same dramatic treatment as the images in which they are embedded.

What all this means, we think, is that it is difficult for local television news—given its tight time constraints and focus on conflict—to cover and explain complicated and interconnected changes in local health care systems. The nature of the medium leads producers and journalists to present imprecise metaphors for these changes: stories of medical mishaps and fraud, for example, that are anecdotal rather than analytical. The challenge is not to change this medium but to devise ways, within the constraints of local broadcasts, to help viewers understand their health care systems better.

CONCLUSION

The pace of change in health care shows no sign of slowing. Readers and viewers look to journalists, in print and on the air, for more than late-breaking news. They look to journalists for reliable and clear guidance about what the latest developments may mean for their health, their finances, and, in some cases, their professional lives and strategies. Researchers can perform a significant public service by helping journalists understand and explain those implications.

Endnotes

1. P. B. Ginsburg and N. J. Fasciano, eds., *The Community Snapshots Project: Capturing Health System Change* (Princeton, N.J.: The Robert Wood Johnson Foundation, 1996).

2. The cross-cutting analyses are collected in a special section of *Health Affairs* (Summer 1996), 7–129. For an encapsulation of the similarities and differences found across markets, see P. B. Ginsburg, "The RWJF Community Snapshots Study: Introduction and Overview," *Health Affairs* (Summer 1996), 7–19.

3. See J. R. Knickman, R. G. Hughes, H. Taylor, K. Binns, and M. P. Lyons, "Tracking Consumers' Reactions to the Changing Health Care System: Early Indicators," *Health Affairs* (Summer 1996), 21–32.

4. E. Tahmincioglu, "Study Finds Managed Care Just Beginning to Penetrate Wilmington," *News Journal* (May 20, 1996), p. D3.

CHAPTER SIX

—∿— Addressing the Problem of Medical Malpractice

Joel C. Cantor
Robert A. Berenson
Julia S. Howard
Walter Wadlington

Editors' Introduction

In the mid-1970s, physicians became concerned about the difficulty of obtaining medical malpractice liability insurance and, where coverage was available, the high premiums. The medical malpractice "crisis" of the 1970s led to legislative changes in many states and to reforms within the insurance industry. Although these reforms seemed to alleviate the situation for a time, it worsened again in the 1980s, raising concern about a new crisis. Although nobody was certain about the extent or the causes of the problem, various legislative and regulatory solutions involving tort reform were proposed.

At the time, few funders were supporting research and demonstrations on medical malpractice insurance. In 1985, The Robert Wood Johnson Foundation began its support of a range of initiatives on the topic. The Foundation's efforts represent a sustained attempt

An earlier version of this article was published in *Health Affairs* (Winter 1994), pp. 230–240.

to understand the problems associated with malpractice and to help foster innovations in the way insurance issues are handled at the state level. Two national programs were supported: the first focused on research to document and explain the situation, and the second supported demonstrations and evaluations of actual reform efforts.

More than a hundred journal articles and reports have been written based on the research undertaken under the two national programs. In many ways, the efforts of those involved in the various projects supported by the Foundation defined a field of research directed at addressing a long-standing problem. In Chapter Six, key people involved in the initiatives synthesize the findings and examine the implications of the Foundation's efforts.

The authors of this chapter were all involved in managing the Foundation's investments in this area. Joel C. Cantor was director of evaluation research at the Foundation until January 1996 and is currently the director of the research division of the United Hospital Fund of New York. Robert A. Berenson, associate clinical professor of medicine at Georgetown University, directs the Foundation-supported Improving Malpractice Prevention and Compensation Systems (IMPACS) initiative. Julia S. Howard is the deputy director of the IMPACS project, and Walter Wadlington, the James Madison Professor of Law at the University of Virginia School of Law, directed the Foundation-supported Medical Malpractice Program.

Despite the press attention given to medical malpractice and the rising cost of malpractice insurance premiums, only recently have researchers focused on documenting the extent of the malpractice problem and finding solutions to it. In the face of firmly held conventional wisdom, many of the research findings are surprising. A Harvard University malpractice study, funded in part by The Robert Wood Johnson Foundation under the Medical Malpractice Program, found that 1 percent of hospital stays in New York state involved medical negligence and that only one in eight of the patients affected by this negligence actually brought a malpractice lawsuit. Moreover, the Harvard study found that the perceived risk of being sued in a given year was three times as great as the actual risk among physicians. Several other studies carried out under the program suggest that doctors' perceptions about their exposure to malpractice liability are simply inaccurate.

In 1985, after a decade of apprehension that harm to patients, and the system of compensation for such harm, could have a severe, adverse impact on physicians and health care institutions, The Robert Wood Johnson Foundation took steps to address these problems by initiating the *Medical Malpractice Program* (MMP). The program was designed to develop and analyze data on medical malpractice and its impact on health care delivery, and to develop strategies for reducing medical injury and adequately compensating medically injured persons. In 1994, the Foundation announced a second major program, *Improving Malpractice Prevention and Compensation Systems,* or IMPACS, which was intended to translate into action the lessons learned in the Malpractice Program by establishing models of malpractice prevention and compensation systems.

As the Foundation has done in many other areas, in medical malpractice it is attempting to effect a change in the system. Because of strong vested interests and systemic inertia, attempts to change a system carry a high risk of failure. If the Foundation's programs *can* bring about changes in social institutions, however, the potential payoff is enormous. The two malpractice programs were created to address the broad failures of current systems. In the view of those who framed the Foundation's malpractice work, the major problems were that:

- Malpractice lawsuits do not provide adequate incentives to correct the vast majority of medical injuries.

- The links between the institutions that address malpractice and the institutions intended to prevent injury and improve health care are weak at best.

- The system is inefficient; only about forty cents on the malpractice premium dollar compensates claimants; the rest goes for legal fees, court costs, and insurer costs.

- Periodically high cost and lack of availability of malpractice insurance have led to problems in access to care for vulnerable populations.[1]

THE MEDICAL MALPRACTICE PROGRAM

In 1987 and 1988, through the Medical Malpractice Program, the Foundation awarded nineteen grants totaling $4.5 million. (Table 6.1 lists these grants and three others that the Foundation awarded through its ad hoc grant-making process during the late 1980s and early 1990s.) At the time that this first program was developed, malpractice premiums had risen to the point of creating a crisis, as they had done in roughly ten-year cycles, but the Foundation staff and consultants could find little in the legal or policy literature to explain these cycles or offer options for addressing the resultant problems. These observations led to the Medical Malpractice Program, which focused on understanding problems and identifying potential solutions.

The Extent of Medical Error and Malpractice

In the 1970s and 1980s, many states passed malpractice legislation even though the legislators had little or no reliable data about the extent of malpractice or the effectiveness of the tort system as a way to compensate victims of medical injury. Two studies supported under the program shed considerable light on this area. The most widely cited of these is the Harvard Medical Practice Study,[2] which, we stated earlier, found that 1 percent of all hospital stays involved negligence and that only one in eight patients injured by negligence filed malpractice claims. This study, based on hospital records from New York state, also found that adverse events (whether or not they were caused by negligent conduct) occurred in 3.7 percent of hospital stays. These rates were similar to those recorded in a study of California hospitals ten years earlier, the basic methodology of which had been followed in the New York study.[3]

The findings of the Harvard study were reinforced by researchers at the University of Chicago, who measured the incidence of error in patient care in three surgical units.[4] Instead of focusing on medical records or insurance claims that had been closed, ethnographers observed hospital units and attended rounds and clinical meetings in which patient care was discussed. Although the purpose of the study was not simply to document the incidence of errors, one finding was that only a small percentage of the patients who were victims of medical error actually brought suit.

Physician and Hospital Practices

Clearly, the best way to prevent malpractice claims is to avoid or minimize the incidence of medical injury. If harm does occur, those responsible should try to mitigate it in a way that is acceptable to the patient. One goal of the Medical Malpractice Program, therefore, was to have the health care and legal communities develop workable responses to medical injury.

Increasingly, health care professionals view the use of protocols, or practice guidelines, as viable tools for improving medical and hospital procedures. Some also see protocols as a means of clarifying the legal standard of care. One study examined the incidence of claims made by patients who went to an emergency room with chest pain or other symptoms but were not treated for myocardial infarction in a timely fashion. Protocols based on this information have been introduced in emergency rooms of military hospitals. Another team analyzed a ten-year database covering some five hundred California anesthesiologists insured by two physician-owned carriers and determined that insurer-introduced protocols had served to reduce claims and thus stabilize liability premiums.

Another study sought to understand whether certain practices or medical providers seemed to be prone to malpractice problems, so that strategies could be developed to reduce the number of events likely to lead to claims. Data on closed claims from a large New Jersey-based insurer were used to identify problem-prone clinical processes in four high-risk specialties: anesthesiology, general surgery, obstetrics and gynecology, and radiology. The investigators found that

Table 6.1   Grants in the Field of Malpractice Made by the Foundation, 1987–1993.

MEDICAL MALPRACTICE PROGRAM ROUND 1

#	Grantee Institution	Principal Investigator	Amount Awarded	Purposes of the Grant
1	American Registry of Pathology	Maj. Frank T. Flannery, M.D., J.D.	$192,094	Prospective study of risk management and practice protocols in hospital emergency departments.
2	Amherst College	James W. Hughes, Ph.D.	95,579	Evaluation of the effect of malpractice reform laws of the 1970s on the number, size, and disposition of claims.
3	University of California, San Francisco	Harold S. Luft, Ph.D.	166,529	Study of the potential use of risk-adjusted liability insurance premiums for hospitals.
4	Harvard University, School of Public Health	Howard H. Hiatt, M.D.	275,937	Study of the incidence of iatrogenic injuries, economic losses, and relationship to malpractice litigation. (Principal funder was the State of New York.)
5	Indiana University Foundation	Eleanor D. Kenney, J.D., M.P.H.	260,094	Evaluation of Indiana's malpractice tort and insurance reforms of 1975.
6	Institute for Medical Risk Studies	Don Harper Mills, M.D., J.D.	231,060	Study of the feasibility and effectiveness of "early warning" systems for malpractice claims.
7	Johns Hopkins University, School of Hygiene and Public Health	Laura Morlock, Ph.D.	285,131	Evaluation of Maryland's 1986 law mandating reporting to a central database of physician disciplinary and tort actions.

8	Johns Hopkins University, School of Hygiene and Public Health	Stephen Teret, J.D.	207,702	Study of early risk factors for malpractice involvement of 1948–1964 medical graduates from Johns Hopkins Medical School.
9	University of Minnesota	Edward Ciriacy, M.D., and Doris Booker, M.D.	296,027	Study of high-risk pregnancies and development of medical-error risk-reduction education for physicians.
10	University of Pennsylvania	Patricia Danzon, Ph.D.	224,650	Study of the economic impact of potential changes in systems of malpractice compensation on physicians and consumers.
11	Private Adjudication Center of Duke University	Neil Vidmar, Ph.D., and Thomas Metzloff, J.D.	284,421	Develop pilot study of alternative dispute resolution (ADR) procedures in malpractice disputes.
12	Stanford University	John P. Bunker, M.D.	200,865	Study of the impact of anesthesiology practice standards on medical outcomes and malpractice claim risk.
13	University of Texas, Health Science Center	Laurence R. Tancredi, J.D., M.D.	300,000	Study of the feasibility of using a list of "accelerated compensable events" as part of a no-fault insurance approach.
14	Vanderbilt University, Institute for Public Policy Studies	Frank Sloan, Ph.D.	225,659	Study of the feasibility of using "damage scheduling" and experience-rated premiums in malpractice insurance.

Table 6.1, continued

MEDICAL MALPRACTICE PROGRAM ROUND 2

#	Grantee Institution	Principal Investigator	Amount Awarded	Purposes of the Grant
15	University of Chicago, Department of Surgery	Thomas Joseph Krizek, M.D.	$290,470	Study of factors that influence patient malpractice-claiming behavior.
16	Maryland Department of Health and Mental Hygiene	Mary G. Mussman, M.D., M.P.H.	87,498	Study of the relative risk of malpractice claims in low-income versus other populations.
17	Oregon Foundation for Medical Excellence	Dennis J. Mazur, M.D.	293,072	Development of a predictive tool to help identify physicians at high risk of malpractice claims or disciplinary actions.
18	Vanderbilt University, Institute for Public Policy Studies	Frank A. Sloan, Ph.D.	299,393	Study of malpractice-claiming behavior and economic outcomes of claims.
19	University of Washington, Department of Family Medicine	Roger A. Rosenblatt, M.D, M.P.H.	295,093	Study of the impact of malpractice systems on access to obstetrical care for poor and rural mothers.

AD HOC GRANTS ON MEDICAL MALPRACTICE

#	Grantee Institution	Principal Investigator	Amount Awarded	Purposes of the Grant
20	RAND	John E. Rolph, Ph.D.	$199,997	Study of using malpractice claims data as a medical care quality-improvement tool.
21	American Law Institute	Paul C. Weiler, J.D.	367,172	Feasibility study of enterprise responsibility for medical injuries, size and disposition of claims.
22	University of Pennsylvania	Patricia Danzon, Ph.D.	49,993	Study of the Swedish system of no-fault medical error compensation.

the claims histories of individual physicians were only modestly useful in predicting whether or not a claim might be filed and thus were of questionable help in targeting physicians for educational intervention or sanctions. On the other hand, the researchers concluded that for an entire system, malpractice data could be used to suggest interventions that might reduce negligence. They suggested that errors involving patients could be averted by such hospital practices as insuring the prompt delivery of test results to physicians.[5]

The majority of malpractice claims stem from harm that occurs to the patient in the hospital. Therefore, risk management programs that are based in hospitals hold potential for limiting substandard care and preventing and controlling claims. Three studies addressed aspects of risk management practices. One grantee explored whether there was a factual basis for concluding that hospital-based risk management programs actually affected the number of claims filed.[6] This study, of forty acute care general hospitals in Maryland during the early 1980s, provides the first large-scale evidence that risk management can help reduce malpractice claims.

Another grantee, in Chicago, addressed ways of developing systems that would bring problems of medical injury to the attention of risk managers as quickly as possible, so that relevant information could be gathered soon after any injury occurred. With this information, the risk managers might be able to resolve a dispute to the satisfaction of the patient without expensive and time-consuming legal proceedings.[7] The project concluded that all hospital medical staff should be involved if reporting on incidence of medical injury is to be effective. This study also pointed to a need for a system that would function more effectively in passing along information about errors to risk managers, patient safety committees, or some part of the hospital administration.

Two other projects, in Oregon and Maryland, addressed the relationship between malpractice and medical credentialing, including state licensing procedures and the granting of hospital admitting privileges to physicians. The researchers in Oregon analyzed an eleven-year database from the state's Board of Medical Examiners to identify physician characteristics and practices that were associated with disciplinary actions and malpractice claims, and the team in Maryland developed guidelines to help hospitals use background information about physicians appropriately and avoid its misuse in the credentialing process. The guidelines were important because Maryland, unlike other states, required reporting of certain malpractice claims and disciplinary proceedings against physicians. Subsequent to this project, the National Practitioner Data Bank, which changed the way information about individual physicians is used in hospital credentialing procedures, was started.

Beyond credentialing or practice protocols, some people have suggested that the perceptions of doctors about legal risk can serve to deter substandard conduct, but others claim that such perceptions can also lead to defensive procedures—diagnostic or treatment measures designed to protect a physician or a hospital from liability rather than to promote patient health. Moreover, several studies under the Medical Malpractice Program suggested that physicians' perceptions about liability exposure are inaccurate. The perceived risk of being sued in a given year was three times the actual risk among physicians studied in the Harvard Medical Practice Study.[8] In a study in Florida, physicians' assumptions about likely malpractice claimants were shown to be unrealistic, and these assumptions varied according to the specialty involved.[9] Three studies supported under the program refute the common assertion that Medicaid patients make malpractice claims more often than others. Studies in the states of Maryland,[10] Washington,[11] and New York[12] revealed that the likelihood of claims from Medicaid patients was no greater than for non-Medicaid patients and in some instances was actually lower.

Whatever the basis for the fears of physicians, the potential result of those fears on doctor-patient relationships and on decisions that affect the cost of treatment or access to medical care can be considerable. The study in Washington state focused first on whether some physicians stop practicing because of a concern about malpractice claims. It found that the attrition rate was small but, because of an already existing shortage of physicians, significant in impact.[13] A further study adding Alaska, Montana, and Idaho found that despite tort reforms, the cost of liability insurance and a concern about the likelihood of being sued continued to limit the number of physicians engaging in obstetrical care.[14]

Understanding and Refining the Legal System

Seven of the projects in the Medical Malpractice Program added significantly to understanding of the effects of conventional tort reforms since the late 1970s and of the functioning of malpractice dispute resolution in general. These projects include studies of the effectiveness of the existing tort system as well as evaluations of tort reforms.

Along with contingency fees and damages for pain and suffering, the civil jury system is among the components of the present compensation system criticized most widely by members of the health care establishment. But one program study found no support for assertions that juries are consistently pro-plaintiff, incompetent, or unjustifiably generous in their awards. The study did find, however, that jurors would like to have greater guidance from judges, particularly with regard to damages.[15]

Fixing the amount of money to be awarded in a malpractice case can be especially controversial. Some critics point to the seeming inconsistency in damage awards, while other critics contend that awards are frequently too high. The distinction between economic and noneconomic loss is of particular importance. These issues were the subject of an extensive Florida study of closed claims for severe birth-related injuries to children and emergency room injuries to adults. In this study, claimants who actually recovered monetary damages received only about 80 percent of the costs that resulted from their medical injuries.[16] The investigators also found that less seriously injured persons received proportionately greater compensation than severely injured persons. They sounded a cautionary note to the effect that the perception that the tort system works poorly may be unduly shaped by publicity about the relatively small number of claims that result in high damage awards.

Indiana was in the forefront of states that enacted broad tort reforms for medical malpractice. Changes included a cap on damages and led to the creation of a patient compensation fund to pay all awards in excess of $100,000, financed by a surcharge on the medical providers' basic liability premiums. Under this system, insurers accepting the first $100,000 of liability in a given case refer the rest of the claim to the compensation fund for settlement. Medical review panels were then created to determine the extent of payment that would be made available under the fund. In an evaluation of the severe-claims experience under the Indiana system compared with that of neighboring states without damage caps, investigators found—to the surprise of some observers—that under the Indiana reforms only a small fraction of claims went before the medical review panels for their determination of liability and that large claims resulted in comparatively generous compensation.[17] The investigators suggest that the

Indiana cap may have inadvertently established what amounted to a no-fault system for large claims.

Some reformers have proposed that medically injured persons must submit their claims to an alternative dispute resolution process, at least initially, as one way to overcome common complaints about the trial system. There are many possible ways to resolve disputes, including arbitration and mediation. The suitability of various procedures in resolving malpractice disputes was examined in one study funded under the program. After analyzing procedural steps taken in malpractice cases that had been litigated in North Carolina, the investigators conducted demonstrations of several approaches, including mediation and arbitration of actual cases that were referred to them through the court system with the agreement of the parties. One innovative alternative was the use of a summary jury trial in specific cases in which the parties agreed to limit the number of factual issues in dispute, the number of expert witnesses, and the overall length of the trial.[18] The parties also agreed to the imposition of a floor and a ceiling on damages. The investigators concluded that the cases most appropriate for summary trials were those in which liability was unclear but potential damages would be great if the recovery was granted.

Researchers in other projects developed or evaluated approaches that would award damages more fairly than the current system and better tailor damages to the needs of medically injured persons. These include development of a plan that would give damage awards precedence in future cases,[19] payment for the future medical services an injured party needs through an insurance contract tailored to specific cases rather than as lump-sum payments,[20] and the introduction of "scheduled" damages—specified compensation for specific injuries—for pain and suffering in medical malpractice awards.[21]

Evolutionary and New Compensation Approaches

In addition to identifying problems that are posed by the way medical malpractice is handled in medical and legal systems and evaluating the major reforms of the 1970s, the program supported work intended to lead to alternatives to the existing systems. Three types of reforms were studied by Foundation grantees.

The idea of a liability system for medical injuries that would rapidly provide fair compensation for certain injuries without need to prove negligence is by no means new. However, past attempts to develop a workable system on such a basis have encountered difficulty in defining what constitutes an appropriate "compensable event." One such approach was developed using a large database of obstetrical injuries on which successful liability claims were founded.[22] The investigators selected the new term *ACE* (for *accelerated compensable event*) to describe the triggering basis for recovery. Although compensation for an ACE would be awarded without proof that it was caused by negligent conduct, experts would generally agree that ACEs should seldom occur in standard medical practice.

ACEs are classes of medical injuries that are readily identifiable and relatively avoidable—in this study, preventable in at least 70 percent of those cases that receive good care. An accelerated compensable event system would not replace the tort system completely, because not all medical injuries would be covered under ACEs. However, the developers of the system estimate on the basis of past claims that between one-half and three-quarters of obstetrical claims would be covered. In concept, ACEs could be extended to much broader classes of medical injuries.

Another project supported by the Foundation examined an even broader reform proposal. The medical malpractice portion of the *Reporters' Study on Enterprise Liability and Personal Injury* for the American Law Institute included a proposal for shifting liability from individual physicians to hospitals or other health care institutions connected with incidents giving rise to claims, except in intentional torts.[23] This approach, called "enterprise liability," would have much greater administrative efficiency than the current system in cases involving multiple defendants and would provide for more-even distribution of malpractice insurance costs that now vary greatly by specialty. Proponents also assert that enterprise liability appropriately reflects changes in the structure of medical practice today, and that it would shift legal responsibility for preventing injuries and improving quality to the institutions that are in the best position to do those things. Such incentives are appealing in light of the findings that the best prospect for reducing injuries is from changes in the system rather than from targeting individual physicians who are at high risk for committing errors.[24] Some who are skeptical about or opposed to such an approach worry that it lessens the deterrent effect of the current tort system, or leads to limitations on physician autonomy.

Finally, no-fault compensation would eliminate one of the most difficult and troubling steps in the present tort system, the finding of fault. Under a no-fault scheme, medically induced injuries are compensable regardless of a finding of negligence. Proponents of a no-fault approach contend that a properly structured plan can provide fair compensation for a greater number of injured parties because of substantial reductions in administrative and other costs. Expenses might be lowered if damages for some types of noneconomic loss were reduced or eliminated. Some suggest that the deterrent effect of the current tort system on substandard care can be (and perhaps has been) substantially replaced by other controls, and that a no-fault system could provide the incentive to reduce all medical injuries. The Harvard Medical Practice Study[25] estimated that a comprehensive no-fault approach would cost no more than the current system but would distribute compensation more broadly and equitably.

Accomplishments and Unmet Aspirations

The most tangible result of the program was a body of research findings: a collection of more than one hundred articles, working papers, books, and reports from the legal, medical, economics, and health policy fields. The success of a program should not be gauged simply by a count of publications, however, but rather by the value and impact of the research reflected in them. In this regard, it is significant that many of the studies provided cornerstones for the current debate among policy makers;[26] others are helping shape new approaches in areas such as risk management and compensation for medical injury (including some with the support of the Foundation-funded IMPACS initiative). Another important accomplishment, although it is a difficult one to quantify, was that the program came to serve as a liaison among researchers from different disciplines—people who had little or no prior contact. In many cases, productive collaboration among program participants continues today.

The program contributed significantly to what is known about the dimensions of medical error, how medical providers view and respond to the current malpractice system, and how the problems of the current system may be overcome. But even the substantial body of research amassed does not address all the important questions raised by policy makers, health care managers, and medical practitioners. Nevertheless, several generalizations can be made from the studies supported under the program:

- Provisions in the health care and legal systems to identify, prevent, and compensate medical injuries are seriously flawed; indeed, the great majority of injuries go unidentified by those suffering them.

- Various stakeholders may view malpractice-related problems differently. Medical providers see the system as arbitrary, for example, while policy analysts emphasize lost opportunities for stronger incentives to prevent injuries and to compensate injured parties fairly.

- Risk management and related mechanisms can be effective, but they are not now sufficiently broad-based and active enough to make a significant contribution to reducing the problem of medical malpractice.

- The best opportunities to prevent medical injuries are in changes to the organization of care rather than in targeting "bad apple" providers.

- Current methods of claims adjudication operate more fairly than many have suggested, but they are slow, expensive, and adversarial and thus compound dissatisfaction in the malpractice arena. Alternative dispute resolution techniques have not been widely adopted.

- There exist promising new approaches to malpractice problems that are ready to be adopted, at least on a demonstration basis.

The most significant obstacle that surfaced early in the Medical Malpractice Program was that many researchers found themselves confronted with unanticipated and often unexplained barriers to data sources, even though the owners of the data had assured them access. In the malpractice arena, more than in other areas of health services, assertions by data providers about confidentiality and potential liability are barriers to research. Generally, claims-related research is limited to closed cases; even so, some malpractice insurers and health care organizations are reluctant to share information. Further research on malpractice requires that keepers of data be willing to open their books.

One area still in need of substantial research is the phenomenon of "claiming behavior"—a special concern, given our knowledge about the relatively small percentage of negligently injured persons who file claims or instigate lawsuits. Also in need of detailed focus is defensive medicine, thus far discussed largely in broad-brush generalizations and a few careful but narrow studies.[27] Other research topics include problems associated with increasing ambulatory care and expanded autonomy of allied health care professionals, the effects of changing practice structures and managed care on fixing liability, special issues of rural practice, the potential impact of outcomes research, and the effects of introducing or withholding new technology or complex procedures on standards for determining liability.

IMPROVING MALPRACTICE PREVENTION AND COMPENSATION SYSTEMS (IMPACS)

As the findings of the research supported under the Medical Malpractice Program came to light, the Foundation shifted its emphasis to applying possible solutions to the problems of malpractice-related systems. In July 1994, the Foundation launched IMPACS, a program that made as much as $6 million available for recipients to prepare, implement, and evaluate demonstration projects. Resources could also be used to evaluate policy changes and demonstration projects that are not funded by The Robert Wood Johnson Foundation. The Foundation, through an external program office and advisory committee, used a combination of two rounds of competitive applications and solicited projects on specific topics that were supported under IMPACS.

As a result of the knowledge gained in the Medical Malpractice Program, the Foundation and its advisers felt that the timing was right for a demonstration initiative such as IMPACS. The history of ten-year cycles in malpractice claims suggested than another crisis period could be expected to begin in the mid-1990s. As in the past, an upsurge in malpractice claims and insurance premiums could be expected to generate considerable interest and political will for reform. It was believed that an interest in reform would spur support for broad demonstration projects.

The Foundation was looking for projects in four broad areas:

1. Providing more appropriate incentives for preventing medical injuries, without giving rise to costly defensive medicine or adversarial provider-patient relationships

2. Incorporating malpractice risk management into quality improvement initiatives of health care organizations

3. Achieving greater efficiency or lower overall cost in processing medical injury claims or compensating injured patients by nonadversarial systems

4. Providing benefits that are more consistent with actual damages for a significantly greater proportion of injured patients

Through the mid–1990s, no new upsurge in malpractice claims or premiums has occurred, and consequently no groundswell of interest in reform projects has emerged. Nevertheless, serious interest does exist, and IMPACS has attracted and is funding a wide range of significant projects.

IMPACS Projects Supported So Far

Table 6.2 lists the projects supported through IMPACS to date. The first two involve planning and feasibility analysis for comprehensive reforms in how malpractice claims are handled in Colorado and Utah. In both projects, members of the Harvard Medical Practice Study team are conducting local versions of the New York study. In both cases, estimates of the incidence of adverse events and malpractice claims are to be made and the costs of the alternative compensation system are to be compared with those of the existing tort system. The design and implementation plans for these two demonstrations also differ in important ways.

In Colorado, staff at the Copic Medical Foundation, the not-for-profit arm of the major doctor-owned medical malpractice insurer in the state, are working to develop an alternative to the tort system. The alternative channels all known cases of medical injury into an administrative system that determines whether a medically related injury took place, and what level of compensation should be granted to injured parties. The system would not require proof of fault before compensation was awarded. The Copic reform model has several advantages over the current fault-based system, at least in theory. First, it provides compensation to a broader range of injured patients and families, and more quickly than the existing tort system does. Second, it is linked to systems of quality improvement and medical discipline, thereby giving clearer and stronger signals for the prevention of future medical injuries. Moreover, such signals reflect medical injuries of all kinds, not just those that result from negligence. Finally, the system is designed to cost no more than the existing tort system, but significant

Table 6.2 Grants Made Through Improving Malpractice Prevention and Compensation Systems, 1994 to Present.

#	Grantee Institution	Principal Investigator	Amount Awarded	Purposes of the Grant
1	Copic Medical Foundation (11/1/94 to 4/30/96)	K. Mason Howard, M.D.	$823,169	Feasibility study for and design of a non-fault-based malpractice compensation system in Colorado.
2	Utah Alliance for Health Care (11/1/94 to 10/31/96)	Elliot Williams, Esq.	729,520	Feasibility study for and design of an enterprise liability demonstration in Utah.
3	Center for Health Policy Research and Education, Duke University (6/1/95 to 5/31/97)	Frank A. Sloan, Ph.D.	526,013	Evaluation of Florida and Virginia no-fault compensation systems for birth-related injuries.
4	Wake Forest University School of Law (6/1/95 to 12/31/96)	Ralph A. Peeples, J.D. Thomas B. Metzloff, J.D.	98,446	Evaluation of court-ordered mediation of malpractice cases in North Carolina.
5	Children's Hospital of Vanderbilt University (1/1/96 to 12/31/96)	Gerald B. Hickson, M.D.	667,291	Demonstration and evaluation of a program of early identification of and response to malpractice risk.
6	Private Adjudication Center, Duke University (2/1/97 to 8/31/97)	Thomas B. Metzloff, J.D. Francis E. McGovern, J.D.	132,732	Planning for a randomized experiment to test mandatory arbitration for malpractice cases in the Philadelphia courts.
7	RAND Corporation (8/1/96 to 7/31/97)	Elizabeth Rolph, Ph.D. John E. Rolph, Ph.D.	177,225	Evaluation of contractual arrangements requiring alternative dispute resolution in managed care organizations.

administration and adjudication costs are redirected into patient compensation.

Copic is creating a detailed design for a model administrative/no-fault system, studying the cost of the reform model, and working with interested parties to refine the model. A number of difficult issues must be resolved as part of the planning process. For instance, how would levels of compensation be determined for specific injuries? What appeals processes would be allowed? And how would the compensation system be coordinated with other sources of funding for medical care and disability, including Medicaid, Medicare, the workers compensation system, and employer-based health insurance? After the model is completed, the proposed reform will probably require state legislation before it can be put into place.

The Utah project is designing a broad-based reform by studying the incidence of medical injury and claims and comparing the costs of a new system with those of the status quo. The model of reform in Utah is different from the Colorado project in several important ways. The former is building on work done under the Medical Malpractice Program, which developed the concept of enterprise liability or responsibility in medical malpractice. In this model, individual doctors are relieved of legal responsibility for medical error, and institutions—most likely hospitals—take on full responsibility. One important advantage of this proposal is that responsibility for preventing medical errors is at a level where systemic interventions can be used. Also in the Utah project, systems for identification of and compensation for medical injury are aligned with quality improvement programs at hospitals. Unlike the Colorado project, the Utah Alliance for Health Care plans to conduct a demonstration of its concept in certain Utah hospitals. As in Colorado, a number of important issues have to be resolved before the demonstration can go forward, such as how to obtain informed consent for patients in demonstration hospitals.

Three other IMPACS projects are evaluations of policies already in place at the state level, and a fourth involves a rigorous study of a new intervention in the Philadelphia area. Frank Sloan and his colleagues at Duke University are evaluating no-fault compensation systems for birth-related neurological injuries in Florida and Virginia. Birth-related injuries are relatively infrequent, but when they do occur they are expensive, and they have been at the center of malpractice concerns in obstetrics nationwide. Florida and Virginia have established funds to compensate families of injured infants without resorting to the tort system. These are currently the only no-fault systems operating in the malpractice arena in the United States, and the evaluators will learn lessons for the broader application of this concept.

A second evaluation project, being conducted at the Wake Forest School of Law, is studying North Carolina's program for court-ordered mediation of malpractice cases. This evaluation compares the program's performance with respect to settlement rates, disposition time, and cost with the performance of the traditional court system.

A third evaluation project, to be run by RAND, is a descriptive case study of the use of alternative dispute resolution, or ADR, for malpractice and coverage disputes in managed care organizations; it is to develop measures of the cost-effectiveness of these programs. The investigators are designing and testing a way to gauge provider attitudes about ADR. The use of ADR in managed care coverage disputes and malpractice allegations may be a way to avoid costly and lengthy lawsuits while still allowing for the fair resolution of claims.

Another ADR effort, to be carried out by the Private Adjudication Center of Duke University Law School, is developing, implementing, and evaluating a court-ordered arbitration model for use in medical malpractice cases. In concert with the state court system of Pennsylvania, the investigators will develop a rigorous examination of the costs and benefits of this type of ADR.

One other project now supported by IMPACS combines demonstration and evaluation. In this project, investigators at Vanderbilt University Children's Hospital are collecting data from multiple sources to identify physicians and clinical situations that receive a high volume of complaints. Prior research by these investigators demonstrated that the volume of general complaints about a physician is associated with an elevated risk of malpractice claims. The information is to be used to develop methods of correcting poor practices. The evaluation will then determine if the program leads to a reduced incidence of malpractice and related claims.

The Future of IMPACS

None of the projects supported to date under IMPACS is far enough along to declare success, or even to generate significant lessons. The researchers are expected to complete their findings in 1997 and 1998. Some of the projects may receive renewal grants for follow-up activities or broadening their work, and there are still several proposals being reviewed that could lead to new IMPACS grants.

CONCLUSION

Within the American health care system, the problem of medical malpractice is not high on the agenda of policy makers; nor is it high among the priorities of those who manage private health care organizations, except for those who must deal with the problem directly. It is natural to ask, then, whether the relatively modest efforts of a private foundation can make a significant difference in this area. Part of the answer is coming as the IMPACS projects play out. Ultimately, though, an answer may not come until a widely perceived malpractice crisis creates the demand for reform. At the very least, much more is known today about the causes and the consequences of malpractice and the functioning of systems for identifying, compensating, and preventing medical injury than was known before The Robert Wood Johnson Foundation launched its initiatives.

Endnotes

1. For a good overview of problems in the system for identifying and compensating medical malpractice, see *Medical Malpractice: Problems and Reforms* (Washington, D.C.: The Urban Institute and Intergovernmental Health Policy Project, September 1995).
2. Harvard Medical Practice Study. *Patients, Doctors and Lawyers: Medical Injury, Malpractice Litigation, and Patient Compensation in New York* (Harvard University Press, 1990).
3. D. H. Mills, J. S. Boyden, Jr., and D. S. Rubsamen, eds., *Report on the Medical Insurance Study* (Sutter, 1977).
4. L. B. Andrews, *Medical Error and Patient Claiming in a Hospital Setting* (Chicago: American Bar Association, May 1993).
5. J. E. Rolph, R. L. Kravitz, and K. McGuigan, "Malpractice Claims Data as a Quality Improvement Tool: II. Is Targeting Effective?" *JAMA* 266 (1991), 2093–2097; R. L. Kravitz, J. E. Rolph, and K. McGuigan, "Malpractice Claims Data as a Quality Improvement Tool: I. The Epidemiology of Error in Four Specialties," *JAMA* 266 (1991), 1–22.
6. L. L. Morlock and F. E. Malitz, "Do Hospital Risk Management Programs Make a Difference? Relationships Between Risk Management Program

Activities and Hospital Malpractice Claims Experience," *Law and Contemporary Problems* 54 (Spring 1991), 1–22.

7. H. Lindgren, R. Christensen, and D. H. Mills, "Medical Malpractice Risk Management Early Warning Systems," *Law and Contemporary Problems* 54 (Spring 1991), 23–42.

8. Harvard Medical Practice Study (1990).

9. F. A. Sloan, P. M. Mergerhagen, W. B. Burfield, and others, "Medical Malpractice Experience of Physicians: Predictable or Haphazard?" *JAMA* 262 (1989), 3219–3297.

10. M. G. Mussum, L. Zawistowich, C. S. Weisman, and others, "Medical Malpractice Claims Filed by Medicaid and Non-Medicaid Recipients in Maryland," *JAMA* 265 (1991), 2992–2994.

11. L. M. Baldwin, T. Greer, R. Wu, G. Hart, M. Lloyd, and R. A. Rosenblatt, "Differences in the Obstetric Malpractice Claims Filed by Medicaid and Non-Medicaid Patients," *Journal of American Board of Family Practitioners* 623–627 (Nov.-Dec. 1992).

12. H. R. Burstin, W. G. Johnson, S. R. Lipsitz, and T. A. Brennan, "Do the Poor Sue More?" *JAMA* 270 (1993), 697–710.

13. R. Rosenblatt, G. Weitkamp, M. Lloyd, B. Schafer, L. Winterscheid, and L. G. Hart, "Why Do Physicians Stop Practicing Obstetrics? The Impact of Malpractice Claims," *Obstetrics and Gynecology* 76 (August 1990), 245–250.

14. R. A. Rosenblatt, R. R. Bovbjerg, A. Whelan, L. M. Baldwin, L. G. Hart, and C. Long, "Tort Reform and the Obstetric Access Crisis: The Case of the WAMI States," *Western Journal of Medicine* 154 (June 1991), 693–699.

15. N. Vidmar, "Medical Malpractice Juries," *Duke Law Magazine* (Summer 1991), 8–12.

16. F. A. Sloan, P. B. Githens, E. W. Clayton, G. B. Hickson, D. A. Gentile, and D. F. Partlett, *Suing for Medical Malpractice* (Chicago: University of Chicago Press, 1993).

17. E. D. Kinney and W. P. Gronfein, "Indiana's Malpractice System: No-Fault by Accident?" *Law and Contemporary Problems* 54 (Winter 1991), 169–193.

18. T. Metzloff, "Reconfiguring the Summary Jury Trial," *Duke Law Journal* 41 (1992), 806–866.

19. J. F. Blumstein, R. R. Bovbjerg, and F. A. Sloan, "Beyond Tort Reform: Developing Better Tools for Assessing Damages for Personal Injuries," *Yale Journal on Regulation* 8 (Winter 1991), 171–212.

20. Blumstein, Bovbjerg, and Sloan (1991).

21. R. R. Bovbjerg, F. A. Sloan, and J. F. Blumstein, "Valuing Life and Limb in Tort: Scheduling Pain and Suffering," *Northwestern University Law Review* 83 (Summer 1989), 908–976.

22. R. R. Bovbjerg, L. R. Tancredi, and D. S. Gaylin, "Obstetrics and Malpractice: Evidence on the Performance of a Selective No-Fault System," *JAMA* 265 (1991), 2836–2843.

23. American Law Institute, *Reporters' Study: Enterprise Responsibility for Personal Injury,* vol. 2 (Apr. 15, 1991), 515–516.

24. Rolph, Kravitz, and McGuigan (1991).

25. Harvard Medical Practice Study (1990).

26. For example, the President's Task Force on Health Care Reform proposed, but later abandoned, enterprise liability—a concept developed in part under a grant to the American Law Institute—as the cornerstone of malpractice-related changes under comprehensive health care reform.

27. G. B. Hickson, E. W. Clayton, C. S. Miller, P. B. Githens, K. Whetten-Goedstine, S. S. Entman, and F. A. Sloan, *"Obstetricians' Prior Malpractice Experience and Patients' Satisfaction with Care,"* *JAMA* 272 (1994), 1583–1587.

~~ Unmet Need in the Community
The Springfield Study

Susan M. Allen
Vincent Mor

Editors' Introduction

In November 1996, the Foundation released a chartbook on chronic illness, noting that ninety-nine million Americans endure the effects of one or more chronic conditions ranging from asthma to Alzheimer's. While the chartbook includes a range of useful statistics describing chronically ill people, the publication also makes clear how much we do not know.

This chapter presents findings from a Foundation attempt to learn more about chronically ill people and the service arrangements for them. The study focuses on a single community, Springfield, Massachusetts. It broke important new ground in measuring unmet needs among chronically ill people and in documenting what happens when their needs for care go unmet. It is unique in that it surveys both people with chronic illnesses and service providers caring for these individuals. The study attempted to understand what the dimensions of a "chronic care system" are, as illustrated by one American community.

Why did the Foundation provide resources for such a study? It hoped that the findings would inform the Foundation's efforts to make grants to improve the organization and delivery of services for people with chronic conditions and would be useful for officials and service providers in Springfield and other cities. It also wanted to look at the value Americans place on support services for people with chronic conditions.

The Springfield Study represents one of a series of investments that the Foundation made four years ago to obtain more information and better data about chronic illness. The most important related project is the 1994 National Health Interview Survey, which was conducted by the federal government with partial support from the Foundation. This survey, whose findings will be released late in 1997, provides information about services, needs, and outcomes of care for chronically ill people.

The authors, Susan Allen and Vincent Mor, are professors at Brown University and researchers affiliated with the university's Center for Gerontology and Health Care Research. They have published extensively on a range of topics related to chronic illness and long-term care and are updating their 1994 data collection to observe how the growth of managed care is affecting service providers and chronically ill individuals in Springfield.

After Congress passed the Americans with Disabilities Act (ADA) in 1990, people with disability were heralded as "the new minority."[1] Historically, however, they have been a hidden minority, restricted to institutions and family homes by both physical and social barriers. But now their visibility is increasing, in part because of trends away from institutional living and also because of ADA-mandated removal of architectural barriers, expanded availability of special transportation, and legal recourse to claims of employment discrimination. As people without disability become more comfortable with having these individuals in their grocery stores, their children's classrooms, and their workplaces, social barriers are also beginning to fall.

The term *disability* is no longer synonymous with people who require a wheelchair to move around; it now connotes a much broader and more diverse population. Defined here as an inability to perform or a limitation in performing routine daily activities or in filling normal social roles because of the impact of chronic illnesses and conditions,[2] disability is fast becoming a focus of health policy concern. There is increasing recognition that the medical model of diagnosis, treatment, and cure that has dominated the structure of our health care system is a poor fit with the needs of people for whom cure is not a possibility but who may live a full life with their disability.

A different model of care and support is called for when the goal is not preventing death but instead managing life with a disabling condition. Regular medical care is important in maintaining health and treating acute episodes, but medical care is only one of a broad array of needs. People with disability may also have social, emotional, and rehabilitative needs, and these vary widely among individuals. Factors that affect specific individual needs include age, availability of financial resources, availability of help from family and friends, and the nature and severity of the disability. One need that many people require is assistance with daily tasks that they cannot perform independently.

How large is this new minority? While estimates of its size vary, results from one national survey indicate that there are more than twelve million people in the United States who need either human or technical assistance in performing routine daily activities. The vast majority of them—approximately 80 percent—live in the community.[3] The assistance they require ranges from help with the most basic life activities, such as eating and toileting, to occasional help with housekeeping and errands. People with cognitive disabilities, such as serious mental illness or mental retardation, often require little hands-on assistance, but they may need supervision and direction in performing tasks themselves.

Since the majority of conditions that cause disability increase with age, we can expect the number of people with disability to grow in future decades. In fact, while people age sixty-five and older now make up 13 percent of the American population, that percentage will climb to 20 percent by 2030 as the full cohort of baby boomers reaches retirement age. Furthermore, the subgroup of elderly people age eighty-five and older, among whom disability is most highly concentrated, is projected to grow most rapidly as medical advances and improved health practices extend life expectancy.

Scientists disagree about the implications of increasingly longer life spans. Some are convinced that longer survival allows time for the onset of other illnesses and conditions, resulting in higher levels of disability among tomorrow's elderly population than among today's. Another theory is that continued medical advances and improved health practices delay disease to advanced ages. Thus, the average American will experience a "compression of morbidity," in which disability is confined to the several years before death. Regardless of which theory turns out to be correct in the end, the combined effects of population aging and extended life expectancy guarantee a substantial increase in the number of people who will require daily support over the next several decades.

The sources of help for this population are largely from family, although both economic realities and women's expanded employment horizons continue to diminish the existing pool of women who stay at home to care for disabled relatives. Highly publicized debates on the future of Medicare, Medicaid, and Administration on Aging funding have rattled nerves not only in the policy arena but also in households throughout the country, and the question of "Who will take care of Grandma?" has become highly politicized. Less visible are nonelderly adults, who, lacking a parallel to the aging system, have even less recourse than Grandma to formal services when family help either is not available or is insufficient to meet their needs.

Given that the structure of reimbursement mechanisms and the health care delivery system revolve around acute care and, to a lesser extent, postacute care, how is this widespread need for assistance being met? More important, *are* these needs being met? And given a scenario of unmet need, what are the consequences of inadequate help?

Medicaid beneficiaries with chronic health conditions made up just 15 percent of the Medicaid population in 1994, yet they accounted for 39 percent of Medicaid expenditures.[4] Policy makers are captivated by the potential of the logic that providing community-based support services such as assistance with daily living tasks will, in the long run, cut costs by offsetting the need for expensive acute care services as well as nursing home care. Underlying this logic is an assumption that there is a causal relationship between not having enough assistance at home and worsening health, the result being crisis management of chronic conditions. To date, however, this assumed causal chain of events leading from unmet need to elevated levels of acute care and nursing home care has not been studied.

In 1992, The Robert Wood Johnson Foundation gave Brown University a grant to study the issue of unmet need for assistance and its consequences among community-dwelling people with disability. At that time, the Clinton administration's quest for health care reform held major promise, since greater attention to chronic care was a focus of the reform effort. Thus, a second interest of the Foundation was to examine the fit between the current system of care and the needs of people with disability as a means of determining what a workable system of care should look like.

Although the President's reform proposals failed, change in the health care system nevertheless is proceeding at a frightening pace. The fee-for-service model that has dominated twentieth-century medical care is fast giving way to managed care, a model emphasizing prevention and health maintenance rather than the treatment of illness. The philosophy underlying managed care is apparently well suited both to controlling health care costs and to maximizing the health of the population. However, the question arises as to how people who already have health problems, many of whom rely heavily on health care services and who require a broad range of supportive and rehabilitative services to continue living in the community, fare under managed care. Can the country adapt the managed care design to fit the needs of people with disability and still achieve cost effectiveness and health maintenance? What features are required to meet both health care and community-living needs? Our study had two major objectives: to determine the nature and organization of the services available to people with disability and to learn the perspectives of both providers and receivers of care.

THE SPRINGFIELD STUDY

For our research, we concentrated all our data collection in one community: Springfield, Massachusetts. This approach allowed us to examine how the culture of the community affects unmet need and what service system is available to the disabled population. We used traditional quantitative survey methods to research the largest of disability subgroups, adults with disability attributable to physical, rather than cognitive, conditions. We randomly dialed telephone exchanges that covered the city of Springfield until we identified 630 disabled individuals. Half of the survey respondents were elderly (age sixty-five and older) and half were working age (eighteen to sixty-four). This quantitative information was complemented by a qualitative study that included people of all ages, representing a range of disabilities. Specifically, we conducted in-depth open-ended interviews with ten members from each of five subgroups: frail elderly adults; children with special needs; and working age adults representing three major disability categories: serious and persistent mental illness, mental retardation, and medical/physical disability. In these interviews, study participants told how they managed disability in daily life, thus adding a depth and richness to survey numbers.

We approached our study of the service system similarly, through a survey of 127 community-based agencies that serve people with chronic health problems within Springfield's city limits and interviews with key agency administrators and providers to learn about their experiences and concerns with providing services to their clients with disability. We also asked these key people their opinions of the major problems with the system as it existed at that time (spring and fall of 1994), as well as their notions of what an ideal system for people with chronic health problems would look like. We used a combination of numbers and stories to evaluate how current arrangements for care and support fit with the diverse service needs of people with chronic conditions and impairments.

THE STUDY COMMUNITY

Springfield has a population of 160,000. Approximately 20 percent of its residents live below the federal poverty line ($10,000 annual income). As of the 1990 Census, 19 percent were African American, and 17 percent were Hispanic, with more than 90 percent of the Hispanics being of Puerto Rican descent. There is general agreement that the next census will reveal increasing diversity in the population, with Puerto Ricans surpassing African Americans in numbers, and other ethnic groups, such as Vietnamese, emerging as the newest minorities. Until recently, Springfield was characterized by distinct ethnic neighborhoods. However, boundaries between neighborhoods are beginning to blur as new immigrants dilute these pools of ethnicity and, simultaneously, sheer numbers create a spillover into other areas of the city. Thus, like urban America in general, Springfield is a mixture of both historically disadvantaged minorities and recent immigrants, and Caucasians make up an ever-shrinking majority.

Once a major manufacturing town, Springfield now relies on the service and educational areas to employ its growing population. Notably, the city's three hospitals are major employers as well as providers of health care for western Massachusetts, and its three colleges attract students from throughout the state as well as its New England neighbors. Thus, unlike similar New England industrial towns, Springfield has not been devastated by the erosion of its manufacturing base. Nevertheless, poverty and urban violence are daily realities.

Massachusetts is a service-rich state bolstered by a generous Medicaid program. Further, the state is progressive in its efforts to adopt programs reflecting a consumer-oriented service philosophy. For example, disability activists consider the Medicaid personal assistance program one of the best in the country. It allows clients with disability to hire, train, and fire their own caregivers. At the time of this study, Medicaid was starting a managed care program, and managed care was rapidly overtaking the private health care sector as well.

A VULNERABLE POPULATION

How are people with disability different from the nondisabled population? To begin with, they are substantially poorer, with fully one-third living on an annual household income of $10,000 or less. Clearly, disability can present obstacles to employment. However, we also know that disability occurs disproportionately among the poorer sectors of our society because of environmental exposures, a high prevalence of trauma, poorer access to medical care, and other factors associated with disadvantaged and marginalized subgroups of American society. So causality goes both ways; that is, disability results in poverty, and the conditions of poverty result in elevated levels of disability.

Disability also presents obstacles to other social advantages. Approximately 40 percent of the people with disability in Springfield have not graduated from high school. The Springfield sample fares poorly in comparison to a national sample of people with disabilities interviewed in a 1994 survey, in which only 25 percent of the respondents reported less than a high school education. An even starker contrast is with the general population of adults, among whom only 12 percent do not have a high school diploma.[5] Furthermore, only 40 percent of the disabled in Springfield are married, and the rate of marriage is not terribly different among those who are working age (44 percent) and those past retirement age (37 percent). We know that spouses are the best line of defense in an illness situation, given their physical proximity and emotional commitment to the person who needs help.

The average person with disability has not one but four disabling health conditions, and this fact suggests both a cumulative effect on physical functioning and, for many, a multiplicity of medical and health-related service needs. The vast majority of the Springfield sample reported at least one musculoskeletal impairment, and two-thirds reported a cardiovascular condition. The most common symptom is pain, experienced by approximately 40 percent of the people with disability and reported as severe enough to have a significant impact on physical functioning.

Technological assistance is important, in that it can increase the extent to which individuals can remain independent of family, friends, and the formal service system. More than half of the people with disability in Springfield now use such technical aids as wheelchairs, crutches, and walkers for mobility—one indication of the effectiveness of the Technology Related Assistance for Individuals with Disabilities Act of 1988.

People with disability rely heavily on medical care because, though not all are "unhealthy," it is undeniably true that people in this group are more susceptible to new illness, and this fact may in turn exacerbate existing levels of disability.[6] Individuals in the Springfield sample averaged twelve visits to a doctor in the year preceding our interview, and just over one-third (35.4 percent) had been hospitalized at least once in this time period. Not quite half (44.7 percent) reported using the emergency room in the past year, with twice as many young and middle-aged adults reporting three or more ER visits as compared with elderly adults; this reflects better access to private physicians among older people through the Medicare program.

NEED AND UNMET NEED FOR ASSISTANCE

Obviously, daily life is made up of routine activities that are necessary for survival. Most of us take our ability to perform these activities for granted. For many people, however, the morning ritual of bathing, dressing, and hair combing presents a challenge that cannot be met without help. These basic life activities are referred to in the medical and research world as activities of daily living, or ADLs.

While ADLs are crucial to survival, more complex tasks such as cooking, shopping, and housework—instrumental activities of daily living, or IADLs—are also critical to maintaining a reasonable standard of community living.

A third area of importance is transportation, particularly as the ticket to medical care, food and other needed supplies, and social and recreational activities. An assessment of need and unmet need for assistance in these three areas—ADLs, IADLs, and transportation—was the primary focus of our population survey.

Nearly three-quarters of the people in our sample (71 percent) report a need for help with at least one ADL. In this study, ADLs include bathing, dressing, transferring in and out of bed and chairs, eating, toileting, and moving around indoors. Not surprisingly, a higher percentage of study subjects (84 percent) report a need for assistance with IADLs—cooking, shopping, light and heavy housekeeping—since the successful performance of these tasks requires a fair amount of exertion, dexterity, and organizational skills. Approximately two-thirds of the people require assistance with transportation; they can neither drive nor take a taxi or a bus by themselves. Unmet need with any given activity ranges from about one-third to one-half of people who need help.

Figure 7.1 illustrates the percentage of people with ADL and IADL assistance needs whose needs are unmet. Some 40 percent of people have their ADL and IADL needs met by their existing support systems; however, the majority of people with needs have inadequate help with at least one daily life activity, and substantial minorities have multiple unmet ADL and IADL unmet needs. Finally, half of the people with transportation needs have enough help, and half do not.

Figure 7.1   Number of Unmet Needs Among Adults with Need for Assistance with ADLs and IADLs.

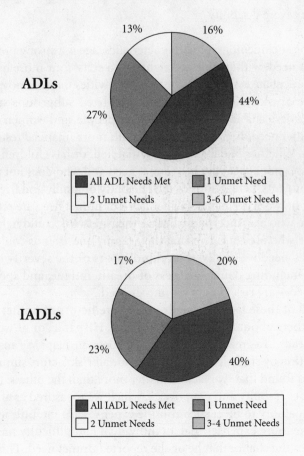

WHO IS AT RISK FOR UNMET NEED?

When we correlate factors that previous research suggests might make a difference in who does and who does not have unmet need, we find that some factors matter a great deal, while others do not. These are the most common characteristics of people who report unmet need, based on the results of our analyses:

• Working age

• Female

• Member of a minority group

• Poor

• Unreliable informal support network

• More severe disability

Among sociodemographic characteristics, age is a strong predictor of unmet need, with people age eighteen to sixty-four more likely to report inadequate assistance in nearly all activities than are people age sixty-five or older. Traditionally marginalized subgroups such as African Americans and Hispanics, poorer people, and women report more unmet need than whites, people with more financial resources, and men. Whether one lives alone, is married, or has children living nearby does not affect who has unmet need and who does not per se, but respondents' perceptions of the reliability of family and friends as a helping network do matter. Higher levels of unmet need are reported by people who are uncertain whether their network could help than by people who are confident that their family and friends could help when they need it. Finally, several indicators of the severity of disability—including pain, shortness of breath, fatigue, and spending days in bed—are risk factors for unmet need.

Are all of these factors equally strong predictors of unmet need? What is there about being a woman, black, Hispanic, or of working age that leads to a greater risk of having inadequate help? We answered this question by statistically controlling for all risk factors simultaneously, and found that two factors matter more than the others: (1) the severity of disability and (2) poverty, which we measured as an individual's inability to meet such routine expenses as rent, utilities, and food.[7] The more expenses that an individual had difficulty meeting, the greater the chance that he or she reported unmet need. This finding makes sense: privately owned vehicles, taxi fare, and privately hired help may not be options for individuals who cannot pay the rent.

The plight of young and middle-aged people with disability is highlighted by the finding about the importance of financial resources, which largely explains the inverse relationship between age and unmet need resulting from more simplistic analysis. Disability for many elderly people follows a life without disability, in which homes were bought, savings were amassed, and pensions were secured. Social Security retirement income is available for most. In contrast, many people who have been disabled from birth or young ages either have never worked or have limited work histories, and consequently have few assets. Subsistence is dependent on Supplemental Security Income or, for those who were disabled after they entered the labor force, on Social Security Disability Income. Neither SSI nor SSDI are as generous as Social Security retirement. Further, Medicare is nearly universally available to the elderly whereas the principal source of medical care coverage in the younger age group is Medicaid, which is not universally accepted by providers, and 15 percent of the younger strata (versus 2 percent of the older age strata) reported no health insurance coverage at all.

The severity of impairment is a major risk factor for unmet need for ADL and IADL help, and this fact suggests that it is most difficult to meet the needs of individuals who require help the most. Both the frequency of occasions requiring help and the extent of help required with specific tasks are undoubtedly greater among the most severely impaired.

We also found that having unreliable helpers leads to unmet need. Clearly, the reliability of the informal helping network is crucial to meeting the needs of someone who cannot perform ADLs and IADLs alone. It is this factor, more than traditional social support predictors such as marital status, having children living nearby, and living arrangement, that is related to unmet need. For example, spouses and other live-in helpers may work, so there are substantial periods of the day when help is not available.

DOES FORMAL SERVICE HELP ALLEVIATE UNMET NEED?

This is a complicated question on the individual level, since the use of formal services may also indicate the severity of impairment, given the stringent criteria that people often must meet to qualify for formal services. However, the higher use of formal support services by the elderly relative to younger adults with disabilities, despite similar levels of illness and impairment, is associated with substantially lower levels of unmet need (see Figure 7.2), suggesting that greater access to formal support services in the home could meet a certain percentage of unmet need in the nonelderly population.

Here again we see younger adults with disability at a disadvantage. Added to the safety net of entitlements available to older adults is the service system for the aged. There exists an array of services available to the elderly that, while far from adequate, may help close the gaps in care: home care programs available under the Older Americans Act, Meals on Wheels, senior centers, and special transportation services, to name a few. Special transportation is now equally available to younger and older people with disabilities through the Americans with Disabilities Act; however, few respondents—only 14 percent—had even heard of the ADA at the time of our survey, conducted three to four years after the act was passed. Finally, there is a certain cohesiveness to the network of services for the aging, as evidenced by centralized information and referral hotlines that may be helpful in meeting needs that arise or in filling gaps in care.

Our study also found a pattern of low use of services and high unmet need among the Hispanic population, whose members with

Figure 7.2.   Age Differences in Unmet Need and Related Formal Service Use.

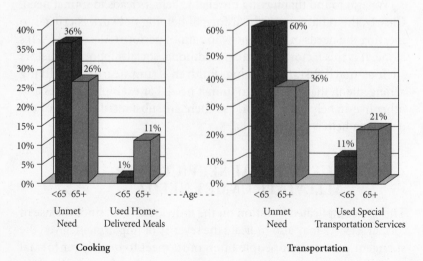

disability used less than half the level of home health aide services (8 percent) relative to whites (21 percent) and African Americans (21 percent) in the study but who reported higher levels of ADL unmet need (67 percent of Hispanics with at least one ADL unmet need versus 52 percent of whites and 54 percent of African Americans). These data suggest that the experience of minorities is not uniform and that the more recently immigrated Hispanics may face greater barriers to getting access to needed services than the more established minorities, such as African Americans. For example, higher proportions of Hispanic respondents than African American or white respondents reported that they did not know of any agencies that provided personal care, household help, or transportation help. A higher use of mental health services among Hispanics in this study also suggests that immigration and acculturation are not without their difficulties.

IS UNMET NEED REAL?

A major objective of the Springfield study was to investigate the first link in a hypothesized causal chain between unmet need for assistance and subsequent elevated levels in the use of acute care service (hospitalizations and emergency room visits), as illustrated in Figure 7.3. We also wanted to provide evidence for our own conviction that individuals' reports of unmet need were valid; that is, that those reports represented a true gap in needed help, rather than simply greed, as some critics have suggested ("Of course people say they need more help. If someone asked you if you need more money, wouldn't you say yes?").

To investigate the validity of unmet need reported by people with disability themselves, we asked respondents whether they had experienced specific, adverse events likely to be associated with unmet need for help with individual ADL and IADL activities and transportation. To be sure that the event in question was related to the lack of help required, we included that attribution in each question, as in, "Have there been times in the past month when you were unable to follow a special diet because you needed help cooking?" Table 7.1 presents the percentage of people with reported unmet need for each activity who responded affirmatively to questions about specific adverse events.

Several negative consequences that we asked about were experienced by the majority of people who had inadequate assistance with the activity in question. Falling due to a lack of assistance in the home, inability to maintain special diets, and inability to eat or drink when

Figure 7.3.   Hypothesized Causal Chain.

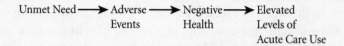

hungry or thirsty may force a transition from community to institutional living. Missing a medical appointment and inability to fill prescriptions or get medical supplies may disrupt compliance with medical regimens and compromise medical management of chronic health conditions. Other adverse events, such as being unable to bathe or put on clean clothes as often as one would like, or not having transportation for recreational purposes, may not have as direct an impact on health status and illness management; however, all are relevant to the ability of people with disabilities to maintain a reasonable quality of life as community residents. In fact, this study found a strong association between experiencing such events and depression, and while the direction of causality cannot be proved from cross-sectional data, it suggests that such adverse events are not inconsequential.

SPRINGFIELD'S COMMUNITY-BASED SYSTEM

We identified 127 agencies that serve people with disability within Springfield's city limits. There are more agencies providing physical, occupational, and speech therapies; information and referral services; mental health services; home health services; and alcohol and drug rehabilitation services than other types of agencies in the community. However, the city's three hospitals (one of them a chronic disease hospital), as major providers of medical care, and government offices, as overseers of various entitlements and benefits, are the largest organizations in terms of number of employees and clientele, serving a broad scope of individuals in both good and poor health. There are three neighborhood health centers available to Springfield residents, one federally funded and the others owned by the area's largest hospital, Baystate Medical Center. These health centers serve primarily minority patients in the community. In fact, for the past several decades, nearly the entire Hispanic population of Springfield has been served by a health center located in the heart of the largest Hispanic community.

Table 7.1   **Proportion of People with Unmet Need Who Experienced Adverse Events in the Past Month.**[1,2,3]

Bathing
   "Unable to Bathe as Often as I Would Like"   73.6%
Transferring
   "Fell While Getting in or out of Bed and Chair"[4]   51.3
Dressing
   "Not Able to Put on Clean Clothes as Often as I Would Like"   28.4
Toileting
   "Wet/Soiled Self"   66.0
Cooking
   "Unable to Follow Special Diet"   38.7
   "Unable to Eat When Hungry"   42.7
Shopping
   "Unable to Fill Medication Prescriptions"   33.3
Heavy Housework
   "Had to Wear Dirty Clothes"   15.0
Transportation
   "Missed Doctor's Appointment"   45.5
   "Unable to Go Places for Fun"   61.1

Notes:
[1] "Past month" refers to the month preceding the actual interview.
[2] The sample for this table includes people who report unmet need for help with the specific activity listed. People who are able to perform the activity by themselves or who have enough help are not included in the denominator.
[3] Respondents specifically attribute adverse events to lack of availability of help.
[4] The time frame for this particular event was "ever," not "in the past month."

Health care and health-related service agencies predominate in this system, although a substantial proportion of agencies—33 percent—report social services or advocacy as their primary offering. These agencies provide senior recreational services, adult day care services, respite services, support groups, employment services, and transportation.

There is a consensus among people who study and work with the disabled population that agencies representing the broad range of health and social services should talk to one another in referring clients to needed services, and that they should share information about the clients they have in common. Communication on the client level should be enhanced by communication at the administrative level in order to advocate for policy change and to plan for improvement in the system. To what extent does this communication actually occur? We found substantially more interorganizational activity on

the client level; for client referral purposes, the average agency communicated with a third of the other agencies in the system and shared
client information with about one-fourth of the other agencies. Communication at the administrative level was far less frequent; agencies
that were engaged in planning activities consulted with only one in
ten of the other agencies on average. A third level of communication,
contractual arrangements, occurred least often of the interorganizational activities studied.[8]

Although the level of interorganizational activity was averaged for
all the agencies studied, in reality a large percentage of all interagency
relations in the Springfield community occur among just a handful of
organizations. Figure 7.4 depicts the core of the Springfield service
system, from which most activity emanates.

Health care agencies dominate this most central of agency groups:
the city's three hospitals are represented, as are two neighborhood
health centers and the largest providers of home care. In addition,
three state agencies, the sources of entitlements, are represented.

The most isolated of the agency groups in the Springfield area—
those operating with the fewest connections to other health and social

Figure 7.4.   Core of Springfield's Community-Based Service System.

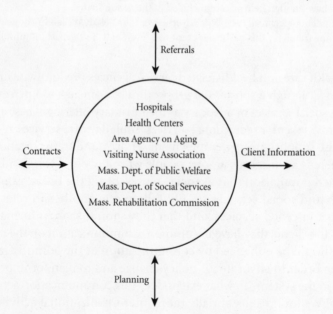

services agencies—are strikingly different from the most centralized group. The isolated agencies are generally likely to be small, for-profit health related service providers, including five agencies providing physical therapy, two providing home care services, and two mental health providers. In addition, this group contains three state agencies that are not directly responsible for coordinating client services, a city government agency, and four social service providers. In contrast to the city's more central agencies, which, for the most part, serve people with a wide range of health conditions, isolated agencies are more likely to serve populations with specific types of conditions, particularly people with physical disability and mental health problems.

Information from the survey of Springfield's adults with disabilities confirms these findings regarding patterns of interagency relationships, at least in regard to referral sources. Forty percent of the respondents reported receiving a referral to community agencies from hospital providers, and 30 percent mentioned at least one referral from private physicians. Given the high level of medical utilization reported by study participants, it is likely that the majority of referrals to services by formal providers are linked to acute events (hospitalizations) or are initiated during emergency room visits or visits to private physicians and clinics. With the exception of the two major home health providers in the city, social service provider agencies do not appear to be major sources of referral to services for this population.

Furthermore, while formal providers predominate in referrals to health-related services such as physical therapy or occupational therapy, referrals from family and friends and self-referrals predominate among services that are more supportive or social in nature—a fact suggesting that it is likely that providers themselves are not sufficiently attuned to the availability of supportive and social services that may be helpful to this population. The lack of integration of health and social services in the system is further evidence that it is oriented to acute care.

SYSTEM BARRIERS TO MEETING NEED FOR ASSISTANCE

The Springfield study was designed to provide perspectives on the service system from both sides of the fence, that is, from service providers as well as the clients served by the system. In both our population and our agency surveys, we asked about barriers to meeting clients' needs. In general, agency providers mentioned system factors, most often related to insurance issues, while our respondents with disability mentioned barriers on the individual level—a lack of knowledge of services, for instance, and a lack of money to pay for them. In our qualitative study of people with all types of disabilities, however, stories about both system- and individual-level barriers to care were raised again and again. We use these experiences to illustrate the problems encountered by people who attempt to use the formal service system to meet their disability-related needs.

Access: Nonreimbursable Services

Although much of the literature criticizing systems of care and support focuses on problems in the organization of service delivery, even the best approaches fail if the full range of services necessary to maintain community living is not available. Services currently accessible through both public and private reimbursement mechanisms have a strong acute care bias that fails to recognize the value of supportive and ancillary services that prevent secondary disability and deterioration of health status.

Neal is a thirty-six-year-old white man who sustained a spinal cord injury when he was struck by a drunk driver. He explains why he moved from Rhode Island to its more Medicaid-generous neighbor, Massachusetts:

NEAL: Well, they, in Rhode Island I find that the Medicaid people there are more geared to when a person needs care, put him in a hospital for the care. But then they complain because the hospital stays are too frequent and too long, yet they don't support home care. It's an infuriating system, you know it's, it's the Medicaid people. . . .

INTERVIEWER: So what are the big differences you see between the Rhode Island system and the Massachusetts system?

NEAL: Here I can get home care. I had one hospitalization when I came here in '88 and I've had no hospitalization since. . . . This state provided my hospital bed, it provided motorized chairs. In Rhode Island, they'd give me a manual chair and say "Fend for yourself. . . ." I just kept getting worse. It was because of the lack of home care I was getting worse and [the] state's unwillingness to leave me in the hospital but unwilling to provide the home care as well. Finally I had enough of it. . . . I said I'm not going back, I left everything in my apartment, my hospital bed, my furniture, my clothes, everything. I just started over again from scratch right here. I said forget it, I'm not even going back to pick up my stuff. [Laughs] Except for my card collection.

Reflected in Neal's story is a basic reluctance on the part of policy makers, providers, and private insurance corporations to distinguish the implications of living through a curable, transient illness as opposed to living with a generally incurable, chronic illness or impairment. Another example is the impact of the failure of most insurance mechanisms to cover dental care, as with Rena, an eighty-two-year-old widow who is reluctant to use special transportation services because she is self-conscious about her appearance. In this case, unmet need is likely to result in increased social isolation for Rena, and possibly, further functional decline:

> Now, I have dentures that I've had a great many years, and they needed attention, but I can't afford new dentures. . . . And at my age, you see a lot of old people toothless, and I would want to be dead if I had to go around like that. You know. . . . 'Cause I had to have one tooth replaced on it. That was $50, at the time which, $50 might not be much to some people, but when you're not working and there's no more coming . . . you know.

Service Limits

People with disability require services that are appropriate to their needs, and they also require that adequate time be devoted to those services. This is particularly germane to supportive help in the home: home health aide, homemaker, and personal assistant services. While some service benefit may be better than none at all, inadequate amounts of a needed service may result in overreliance on the informal support network, or, in the absence of informal support, unmet need for a particular service. Both scenarios—strain on the informal support system and the experience of unmet need—may threaten the viability of community residence.

Dave is a thirty-year-old African American with quadriplegia incurred in a car accident twelve years before our study. Even the fifty hours of attendant care per week allotted through the Medicaid personal assistance program is not enough to meet his needs. He explains his frustrations in having to live with his mother because he needs to be turned every two hours:

INTERVIEWER: And then, you have the people come in the evening, didn't you say?

DAVE: No. Because my mother's here.

INTERVIEWER: So your mom comes and helps you when you get turned at 4:30?

DAVE: Yeah, yeah. . . . That's what's stopping me from being more independent and having my own place. Because, and that's one thing, because they don't supply enough hours for me, to actually, I would love, I mean, thirty years old, and still living with your mom. You know? I mean, there's nothing wrong with my mother, but still I'd like to be a little bit more independent.

Dave's dilemma is at the heart of the frustration felt by disability activists who question why the system guarantees people with disability the right to equal employment opportunities but often does not provide the services they need to get up and get dressed in the morning. While the goal of the ADA is to maximize opportunities for independent living and participation in the mainstream, Dave's story illustrates the obstacles that remain to achieving such goals.

Emily, an elderly white woman recovering from a hip fracture, notes the effect of recent cuts to her homemaker program:

She comes for one hour and forty-five minutes, which does not permit a human being to really do what is necessary. She happens to be a good worker and a very good person and we have a good relationship. She does my laundry . . . which is time consuming. Um, she scrubs my, my tub. Which I can't do. She does the floor. She vacuums. She dusts and polishes. . . . They cut the hours from three hours, which was adequate . . . to one hour and forty-five minutes . . . but it does fit their budget, so everyone gets a little bit, very little.

Emily says she attempted to do some undone tasks herself, nearly falling again and risking further injury.

Lack of Continuity in Service Delivery

A chronic illness may consist of numerous phases, with stages of greater or lesser need for acute care, rehabilitation, and home-based support. The optimal management of chronic illnesses and conditions is clearly dependent on the ability of the system to provide smooth transitions to accommodate changing medical and social needs.

A lack of continuity may be due to the acute bias of insurance coverage, to poor coordination of care transitions, or to both. Some elderly participants reported problems related to coordination of care, which resulted in inadequate or nonexistent home health services after they moved from hospital to home. Ed and Gene, both elderly men who lived alone, and both of whom reported having a social worker or a case coordinator, received no help after their hospitalization. Gene, who returned to a hospital and later a nursing facility during our study, told us:

> They take me home, and dump me on the couch. They were supposed to send 'em back up for my medicine and stuff. And no one ever showed up. So, then I'd end up back in the hospital. . . . If I coulda got somebody to stay in with me for my meals and medicines and stuff, before I got too bad off, I mighta been able to make it. But I couldn't get nobody . . . should've been done before, before it was too late. . . . There's no way I'm going to be going home. I can't hardly get outa bed.

Ed's story was similar:

> And then, at the hospital, you know, they're mean. . . . You see now, when you're poor like this, you know what, they sent me back home. I was livin' alone. But they gave me so much goddamn dope there, I mean the pain pills, that I did feel pretty good. . . . So I came home by myself, and it's kinda tough . . . a man that sick should never never never be sent home alone.

A second type of transition requiring different constellations of service is the transition from one stage of the life course to the next. This issue is particularly relevant for people with mental retardation, who lose access to primary care physicians knowledgeable about their special health and social needs as they transfer out of the care of pediatricians.

Donald is a twenty-five-year-old Caucasian with Down's Syndrome who lives with his parents. According to his mother:

> Donald had a breakdown about two years ago. Right after he left school, that was a *big* transition. Boy, if mothers ever want to pick my brain, the biggest thing I'll tell them is *prepare* for that change [turning twenty-two]. It's physically, emotionally, and socially a very difficult change. School structures their life for so many years and then on their twenty-second birthday, right in the middle of the school year, it doesn't make any difference whether they. . . . On March 26, three years ago, his transportation stopped and his schooling stopped, on that day. . . . Boy, you are not . . . the client nor the family are not ready for that change. That change is just emotional. . . . And it's at a difficult time in their lives. . . .

Lack of Service Integration

The funding of health and social service benefits for people with disability is fragmented among public, private, and voluntary sources, and the result is a system lacking in accountability for individual clients. In other words, current systems provide not a protective blanket of health and social services but rather patchwork quilts, with the size and the adequacy of each individual quilt depending on the number and the size of the patches for which one is eligible. Furthermore, the structure of the system, combined with professional ideologies and issues of turf, results in little guarantee that an individual's attempts to get from one service to another will be facilitated by formal care coordinators.[9]

The parents of children with special needs are most eloquent about difficulties in coordinating the services they need, often reporting that their children were assigned several case coordinators, each one from a specific agency and therefore unable to make connections to all the services required by their children's needs. Many parents took on the coordinating role themselves. Rick, one of the children's fathers, told us:

> It seems like a lot of things are out there, but it's not coordinated. A lot of the information doesn't get out. We went to this parent conference on early intervention last year. . . . They offered just a packet of information on SSI and other services that are available to the area. . . . You know what would be nice? To have somebody there do a case

management service to coordinate all the stuff for you, or if you couldn't hire someone to do it, then have the government or some state agency pay you to do it, because it can take up a lot of time.

Provider-Driven Services

Central to the disability rights movement is the rejection of the belief that medical care providers best know the needs of people with disability. Activists and advocates promote instead a consumer-directed model of service delivery in which clients, not providers or clients' family members, determine what services are required to meet the clients' needs. This sentiment is echoed by our study members, who complain that the services available to them are often not particularly helpful because they are ill-suited to accommodate the preferences and needs of clients. A woman named Frances describes her interaction with her home health aide:

> I told her not to use so much stuff in the bathroom, because it choked me and it was expensive. . . . She said, "You don't have to tell me what to do, I know what to do. . . ." I went through hell the day before with my sister dying, I said, "You could have a little consideration for somebody," and she's going, making like, mocking me. You know what I mean? I mean this is aggravating, and when you're old, and you don't feel good, this doesn't make your health, I don't think, any better.

Frances's lack of power in negotiations with her home health aide was clear:

> So she says to me, "If I don't work for you, they'll get me somebody else. . . . All I got to do is call up the agency supervisor."

Some service agencies in the Springfield area reported total agreement with the disability movement's service philosophy and its goals of client preference and independence. For example, several of our study participants were connected with programs that were sponsored by the Department of Mental Health and that emphasized an individualized and client-directed approach to service delivery. One of these, a program called AIM (Alternatives to Institutional Maintenance) provided assistance with community placement and daily living. Like the Medicaid personal assistance program, these programs for the mentally ill supported the independent-living model of service delivery, in that participants were "consumers" of mental health services and were using the services to strive toward goals they determined for themselves. The director of AIM outlined the service goals of her program:

> We try to help people be more autonomous, to live on their own, to figure out what they want. And, within reason, to help them get that. Some people need support in learning to use public transportation. Some people need us to help them set up a savings plan 'cause they want to buy a car. Some people want to have a job. . . . You could interview twenty-one different consumers, and you would get twenty-one different things that they want.

Service Gaps

Whereas there were some discrepancies in the perceptions of barriers to the use of services among the providers and the consumers, the perceptions of service gaps were quite congruent. Three service gaps reported most often by our agency survey respondents, and often reflected in the narratives of participants, were housing, transportation, and productive activities, such as vocational training and employment. A fourth gap, mentioned by people in every disability group represented in our study—but by only one agency—was the lack of social and recreational opportunities.

Housing issues came up most often in relation to people with mental retardation who were on waiting lists for residential placement. Some people had been waiting for four years at the time they were interviewed for our study. This may be the result of the narrowing of eligibility criteria for services in this population, with persons who had mild retardation either not qualifying for services at all or qualifying only for waiting-list status. It seemed that such status was equivalent to disconnection from the service system. Barbara's son, Peter, has been on a waiting list for a group home for three years, despite the fact that he has occasionally injured his mother when he becomes unmanageable. Peter's sister and her boyfriend, both of whom are also mentally retarded, are cared for by Barbara as well. She explains:

> Well, we really would, are trying to get him into a halfway house, so that he can live away from home. He's pretty rough . . . and I'm getting old . . . I would like to see Peter live independently . . . you know,

if something happens to me . . . and I want maybe a little more freedom myself.

Stories abounded about inadequate, unreliable, and altogether unsatisfactory transportation services in the Springfield community, despite the fact that public transportation authorities were increasing the number of special transportation vans to meet a Disabilities Act mandate. The act requires public transportation lines to provide regular bus routes for people with disability. Clients must meet certain criteria to become ADA-certified for these services, but, once certified, transportation authorities must respond to all requests for rides, given twenty-four–hour notice. Nor are services confined to worthy errands such as doctor's appointments; requests can be made for any reason.

The ADA mandate initially created transportation wars between the frail elderly, who were accustomed to the free use of the city's transportation vans, and younger persons with disability, who now competed with and at times bumped those elderly who were not sufficiently impaired to become certified under the terms of the ADA. One elderly woman mentioned her frustration at being made late for a doctor's appointment to accommodate a younger person's whim to get a pizza. However, subsequent visits to the city revealed that the transportation wars had been downgraded to occasional skirmishes as the transit authority met its full ADA implementation deadline of 1995.

The need for productive activity was a particular issue for people with cognitive disabilities in our study. All study subjects with mental retardation who were working held jobs in Goodwill or state-supported workshops. The programs tended to consist of repetitive work, sometimes amid considerable noise and other disruptions. Subjects and caregivers we interviewed reported no knowledge of other services to use for employment or productive activity. Ella, Gene's mother, told us how this situation affected her son's life:

> It is very difficult for him to sit all day in the same position and do the same job. That's the way most of the programs are set up. . . . Sunshine Village does have some off-site, small-group, contract-type work that we would like to [steer] him in that direction. But he would start again in the large, production-type ring. And he really finds that very difficult. . . . He can't handle noise, he can't handle any confrontation . . . and there [in the large group] are some clients that are very disruptive and loud, and that kind of thing.

Eddie, a man with mild mental retardation, had been seeking part-time employment for quite some time, since he knew that a full-time job was out of the question for him. Since his disability was not severe, he was wait-listed for an employment opportunity:

> I ain't worked in two years. All I could find is full-time job, I can't find no part-time job. All they got is full time and I can't work it. . . . [The case manager] told me he ain't got no funds, no money or nothin'. Ain't got no funds. . . . I call him about three days a week. . . . I talk to him about something like that . . . he ain't got nothin'.

People with mental illness also expressed the desire to work. However, some found that the services they used to find paid employment were a poor fit. Jonathan, who was a college student before he was hospitalized because of schizophrenia, tried to use Department of Mental Health employment services to reenter the workforce:

> I'd love to have a job. . . . I could do a factory job. . . . I figured they'd just ease me into some place you know, like we have these connections . . . [but they don't have] close contacts, they don't know anybody there, or you have to have a degree, or it's a million miles away, you don't have a car. . . . I just thought I'd had enough . . . so I don't need the [DMH] services.

A number of study members with severe mental illness spent their weekdays at the Lighthouse, a clubhouse model of service delivery that provides jobs in the form of employment within the organization as well as job training for positions in the community. The Lighthouse also serves as a place to go for socialization activities. However, it is a Monday through Friday operation, leaving club members on their own for the weekend. Rob, a young man who has been unable to hold a job for quite some time, tells us:

> Weekends are a hard time for me. There's nothing on TV, just wind up lying around, basically doing nothing. . . . I'd like to go out once in a while, eat out. . . . Activities are a big, big problem for us. 'Cause we just don't know what to do, and we have limited money. . . . We want desperately to have something, we get nothing. . . .

Problems of living with unrelieved boredom and loneliness are not confined to the cognitively impaired. Here's what Gene, an elderly gentleman, told us:

My friends, more or less, and a lot of 'em, oh, 80 percent of 'em are dead. . . . Ed's dead. . . . There's no word in Webster's Dictionary to describe loneliness. I think it is the worst word. The worst thing going. Like I told ya, sometimes I'm home on the weekend, I don't go out. One day, I told my brother I was in here for ten days, of course, weather, too, has a lot to do with it. And I thought I was gonna die of loneliness . . . and that's the worst sickness going, you know.

Socialization with nondisabled persons was rare for a substantial number of those in our study. For example, a young physically disabled man laughingly referred to "my one ambulatory good friend." When asked about interacting with nondisabled people in the community, Terry, another person who became disabled in adulthood, shared his concerns:

[I've] become a lot more withdrawn, you know? . . . I don't want to use the term "afraid," but you know, maybe like right now I don't know if people are accepting me or not accepting me because of disability or because of something else. You know? If they weren't accepting me not because of disability, that's all right. But if they're not accepting me because of disability, then that would bother me.

It is clear from these narratives that several factors contribute to social isolation for these people. Predominant among these factors are a lack of access to opportunities available in the community and perceptions of others' attitudes toward their disability.

THE BOTTOM LINE

This snapshot of adults with disability living in one midsize American community, and their relationship to the community-based service system, delivers a clear message: the status quo does not work. Levels of unmet need for assistance with daily living tasks are substantial, and we were able to capture at least some of the immediate consequences resulting from inadequate help. The stories told here cannot begin to capture the poor quality of the lives of these individuals, many of whom lack the services and financial resources to meet any but the most basic needs. Furthermore, these people were service-connected, and therefore not among the most isolated or needy.

Two things are clear: while use of the formal service system can alleviate unmet need to a certain extent, the shortcomings of the system often create situations that should not occur. Service gaps, service limits, lack of continuity, poor coordination . . . the litany goes on. As policy makers and program developers ponder how to rework managed care for the healthy into managed care for the disabled, we hope they have the appropriate goal in mind: meeting the full range of needs of this most vulnerable of populations. And if it is done right, cost containment may well follow.

Endnotes

1. J. P. Shapiro, *No Pity: People with Disabilities Forging a New Civil Rights Movement* (New York: Random House, 1993).
2. M. A. Pope and R. A. Tarlov, *Disability in America: Toward a National Agenda for Prevention* (Washington, D.C.: National Academy Press, 1991).
3. General Accounting Office, *Long Term Care: Diverse, Growing Population Includes Millions of Americans of All Ages,* GAO/HEHS–95–26 (Washington, D.C.: author, November 1994).
4. General Accounting Office, *Medicaid and Managed Care: Serving the Disabled Challenges State Programs,* GAO/HEHS–96–136, Washington, D.C.: author, 1996).
5. L. Harris and Associates, *N.O.D./Harris Survey of Americans with Disabilities. Report to the National Organization on Disability* (New York: author, 1994).
6. G. DeJong and R. Brannon, "Trends in Services Directed to Working Age People with Physical Disabilities," in S. Allen and V. Mor (eds), *Living in the Community with Disability: Service Needs, Use and Systems* (New York: Springer, forthcoming).
7. S. Allen and V. Mor, "The Prevalence, Determinants, and Consequences of Unmet Need for Assistance with Daily Living Tasks Among Older and Younger Adults with Disability," *Medical Care* (forthcoming).
8. J. Banaszak-Holl, S. Allen, V. Mor, and T. Schott, *Subsystems within Community Agency Networks: Barriers or Channels to Service Provision?* unpublished (1996).
9. S. Allen, "People and Systems: Assessing the Fit," in S. Allen and V. Mor (eds), *Living in the Community with Disability: Service Needs, Use, and Systems* (New York: Springer, forthcoming).

—∿— **Unexpected Returns**
Insights from SUPPORT

Joanne Lynn

Editors' Introduction

Chapter Eight presents selected findings and lessons from a large, multiyear research-and-demonstration project that investigated the care provided to critically ill hospitalized patients at the end of life. SUPPORT, as the study was called, was motivated by a sense that services provided to people who are dying overemphasize heroic, high-tech innovations at the expense of caring and comforting.

Although the motivation was simple, it turns out that the problem is not. This chapter describes the complexity of addressing the issue of what services ought to be delivered at the end of life and the difficulty of changing norms and practices in the world of medicine. The chapter emphasizes that it is not so simple even to identify what we mean by "the end of life."

Considerable effort was given to ensuring that the project's findings would receive widespread media attention. As a result, the project seems to be provoking the wide-ranging and, we hope, sustained debate that is necessary to make progress on this problem. The study was reported in cover stories of weekly newsmagazines and many

articles in noted academic journals. The researchers have been bar-
raged with requests to appear on television and radio shows to discuss the implications of the findings.

The findings from the demonstration project at the core of the study
were negative: the interventions did not achieve the goals expected.
However, the large investment by the Foundation—which has totaled
approximately $29 million to date—may have other payoffs. The find-
ings clarified that changes in care at the end of life are not going to
happen with marginal adjustments in the way we organize services. It
takes a much more sustained effort on many fronts to refocus priorities
for the care of the critically ill. Changes in social norms, professional
values, and social priorities all need to be part of the solution.

SUPPORT suggests another lesson for a philanthropy that uses some
of its resources to support research and analysis. The project was
expensive in part because of the detailed, high-quality data-collection
effort designed to measure outcomes associated with different interventions. This dataset is providing a range of collateral payoffs as the
research team explores the data. For example, an important study published by some members of the team raises serious questions about the
efficacy of the Swan-Ganz catheter, a common intervention to monitor
cardiovascular function in critically ill patients in hospitals. Thus, investments in quality datasets can lead to important research beyond the
questions that motivated the data collection.

The chapter was written by Joanne Lynn, who is an Emily Davie and
Joseph S. Kornfeld Foundation Scholar and the director of the Center
to Improve Care of the Dying at George Washington University. Lynn
codirected SUPPORT with William Knaus, who is now chairman of the
Department of Health Evaluation Sciences at the University of Virginia.
The insights presented emerge from the collaborations of a national
team of investigators that made the project happen. Lynn was involved
in the study from the beginning, and she continues to work on research
and medical innovations to improve care of the critically ill. As with
many of the other chapters in this book, Lynn's chapter just scratches
the surface of the many findings that have emerged from this complex
study. We urge interested readers to seek out some of the many articles cited in the references.

T he Study to Understand Prognoses and Preferences for Outcomes and Risks of Treatments, or SUPPORT, collected a remarkable variety of data on 9,105 very sick hospitalized patients, identified problems in their care, and tried and failed to correct those problems. SUPPORT assembled the most comprehensive database to date describing very sick hospitalized patients and especially the care of those who die. Why the project failed to correct the problems with care remains an intriguing and enlightening focus of inquiry. This chapter provides an overview of the development and methods of the project and then examines an array of issues that SUPPORT helps to illuminate, often in unexpected ways. Some of what is reported here is straightforward, noncontroversial data; some is more speculative and challenging.

The early 1980s were marked by concerns over the cost of health care, culminating in such reforms as the use of diagnostic-related groups in the Medicare program and by highly visible controversies over patients' rights, especially at the end of life.[1] Fueled by a series of personal experiences that affected the leadership of The Robert Wood Johnson Foundation, a concern arose at the Foundation that elderly, fatally ill persons were likely to be vigorously treated in intensive care units, at great financial cost and suffering, even if their families objected. In 1985, the Foundation convened a meeting to consider these issues. After that meeting, the Foundation staff invited a few researchers, including William Knaus and me, to write a letter about what could be done to understand and improve care of critically ill persons in hospitals. This initiated three years of correspondence, meetings, and piloting that gradually shaped what became the SUPPORT project.

The project was carried out in two stages, with a first stage of description (1989–1991) and the second intervention (1992–1994). In planning for the first phase, the team overseeing the study at George Washington University made a number of decisions:

• Since more accurate and usable prognostication might have an important role in the treatment of critically ill patients, we decided that the study populations should be ones for which the physiology was relatively well understood. We settled on nine specific diagnoses: acute respiratory failure, multiple organ system failure with sepsis, multiple organ system failure with malignancy, chronic obstructive pulmonary disease, congestive heart failure, chronic liver failure, nontraumatic coma, colon cancer, and lung cancer.

• We determined to seek much of the important information through personal interviews. This, we decided, would be the best way to determine the functional status and cognitive ability of the patients, learn their preferences, and understand the appropriateness of intensive treatment (for example, knowing whether the patients and families understood and desperately wanted that treatment, or whether they were uninformed, confused by their options, or opposed). Proposing substantial interviews of the very sick and their families was unusual, and many observers thought it unlikely to succeed. Piloting showed, however, that patients and families were generally easy to interview, some even grateful that research was under way. As one might expect, resistance from busy physicians to intrusive and time-driven interviews was more of a problem.

• We decided to concentrate on a small number of hospitals in order to collect high-quality information intensely, but we also wanted them to be diverse and reasonably representative of national experience. In order to enroll enough patients to warrant the infrastructure, hospitals would usually have to have more than five hundred beds, and in order to be familiar with managing research and protecting subjects, they would have to be hospitals with teaching and research functions.

The Foundation staff was closely involved throughout. One of their strong contributions was the insistence that we be committed to addressing problems the study identified; this was made a condition of participation for the eventual collaborating group. The study was perceived as being quite risky, with many more ways to fail than to succeed; funding was always for short time periods and contingent upon showing that some aspect of the study could be carried out.

In 1988, we issued a request for proposals to all American hospitals with teaching programs. The full application was completed by fifty-five hospitals; eleven were visited and five were selected.[2] The study was fielded in June 1989, and it enrolled patients for two years.

Nearly every patient with one of the nine diseases at a defined advanced stage was enrolled.[3]

Phase I

The first phase described these serious illnesses, their outcomes, and the decision making that might shape their course. Valid, well-calibrated models to predict survival time[4] and serious functional disability[5] were major accomplishments of Phase I. We also showed that we could get high-quality data at every stage: identifying patients; interviewing patients, families, and physicians; reviewing medical records; and managing a very complex data collection and database.

By the end of Phase I, the kinds of problems that might be worth trying to improve were becoming clear.[6] Decision making was often far short of ideal. Physicians did not know what patients wanted with regard to resuscitation, even though these patients were at high risk of cardiac arrest. Orders against resuscitation were written in the last few days of life. Most patients who died in the hospital spent most of their last days on ventilators in intensive care. We had not expected to find the high levels of pain that were being reported, especially in non-cancer illnesses. Except for the comatose, more than half of the patients with any one of the nine diseases were reported (by the patient or a family member) to have substantial pain, and we felt obliged to make reducing pain a target of the intervention.

Phase II

When Phase I finished enrollment, in June 1991, we faced substantial pressures to design Phase II quickly. The staff and the infrastructure at the five sites were established and effective, but costly. Some downtime allowed completion of follow-up, cleaning up records, and doing validation and reliability studies, but we could not afford to keep the teams together for long. Thus, we decided on an intervention by midsummer and piloted it in November. Enrollment for Phase II started in January 1992 and ran through January 1994.

The intervention included frequent reports from the computer model for prognostication and reports from interviews with patients and their families. It was anchored, however, by specially trained and committed nurses who spent all their time counseling patients and families, convening meetings with physicians and others, eliciting preferences, making plans for future contingencies, and ensuring that the best possible information about prognosis and preferences was available to the care team. These nurses managed to carry out the intervention with grace, forcefulness, and timeliness. They had some communication with all of the intervention patients' physicians; prognoses were delivered for 94 percent; patients or families met with the SUPPORT nurse in 84 percent of the cases, and, for patients who stayed at least a week in the hospital, the SUPPORT nurses averaged six visits.[7]

In shaping the intervention, we wanted to be absolutely sure that any benefit we claimed was really associated with the intervention itself and did not arise from changes with time or simply from the changes that people make when they are being studied. This required that there be a set of concurrent controls—people who were not receiving any intervention. Since there were substantial variations in every potential target of the study, controls would have to be established at each hospital.

We realized that it is hard to induce change, so we were willing to try a multifaceted approach. The institutions, through their institutional review boards, were concerned about the disruptive potential of the intervention. They relied on the attending physician to arbitrate whether a patient could be involved, and this decision required that we recruit all possible attending physicians. The institutions saw the proposed intervention as being like an unproved drug, and they required that reports from the prognostic models, the interviews, and the nurse's involvement be prominently labeled as research material. Thus, reports could not be given directly to the patient or the family.

In order to avoid contamination between the control and intervention patients, the patients of any one physician would either all have to have the intervention or all not have it. Since physicians were working in various collaborations, often concentrated in certain sites at the hospital, we had to allocate the intervention by physician groups. In other words, all patients of intensive care physicians at one hospital had to have the intervention, while all patients of intensive care physicians at another hospital did not. Otherwise, the commonplace practices of sharing patient management, rotating attending coverage, and cross-covering would lead to contamination.

Within these constraints, we tried to have the most aggressive intervention possible. We held focus groups of physicians to assess the merits of various possibilities. Those groups and a review of the literature, including the law, showed that many doctors claimed to be eager to improve care and decision making for the seriously ill, but they maintained that improvements took too much time and they often did not have the needed information about prognosis and patient preferences. We set out to reduce those time-and-information barriers.

As we geared up to initiate Phase II, we completed an ancillary study of the prevalence and outcomes of illnesses severe enough to be likely to qualify for enrollment in SUPPORT (but including people who did not come into the hospital or otherwise did not qualify), using the population around the Marshfield (Wisconsin) Clinic, one of the participating sites. This study showed that most patients with SUPPORT-like illnesses were not coming into the study, and that those who were not were disproportionately old, disabled, and cared for at home or in a nursing home.[8]

We also noted that our age range was lower than the national range for dying generally, and that the study actually had few patients in advanced old age. In order to capitalize on the unique opportunity offered by having an extensive data-collection arrangement in these hospitals, we added a descriptive study of the hospitalized elderly in 1994. This addition was called HELP, the Hospitalized Elderly Longitudinal Project.

The intervention phase was monitored for adverse effect by an external review committee, but otherwise data were blinded until follow-up was completed, in June 1994. During Phase II, the hospital staffs and the patients and families generally liked the intervention nurses. Two hospitals moved to continue them at the end of funding. The nurses themselves were a little skeptical that there would be an effect on the five issues chosen for formal evaluation of the effect of the intervention, though they were sure that their work was appreciated by all concerned and that it was valuable. Once the data were unblinded, it was clear that the intervention had not improved any of the five targeted problems:

1. The timing of a "do not resuscitate" (DNR) order

2. Accord between patient and physician about DNR

3. Time spent in an intensive care unit (ICU) in a coma or on a ventilator before death

4. Pain

5. Resource use[9]

INSIGHTS ABOUT DYING

Although SUPPORT was designed mainly to describe and improve outcomes and decision making regarding serious illness in hospitals, it also reported on the largest group of dying patients ever described in American hospitals. This is not a cross-section of dying; patients in SUPPORT had an established and diagnosed serious illness; they had been hospitalized and survived forty-eight hours; they were younger than the population's average age for death, and they were in large teaching hospitals. Nevertheless, describing their experience has been important. They do account for 19 percent of the adult deaths in these hospitals, but just 3 percent of the admissions.[10] About one-fourth of them had serious pain while they were hospitalized; the families of those who died reported that, of the half who were conscious at all in their last few days, one-half of them had moderate to severe pain most or all of the time.[11] Pain was spread across all diseases, not just cancer.[12]

While half of the SUPPORT patients died after more than one week on a ventilator in an ICU,[13] only 14 percent had had a resuscitation attempt when death came.[14] Surely that is an improvement upon the widespread utilization of cardiopulmonary resuscitation in such situations a decade or two ago, but it still is troubling. To be in SUPPORT with congestive heart failure, for example, a patient had to have too little reserve to walk around in a room, even while on maximum therapy. These are patients whose hearts are exceedingly unlikely to sustain circulation after any further injury, yet almost one-fifth of them received resuscitation at death. CPR was tried on about 5 percent of the patients with widespread lung or colon cancer.[15] Surely these rates would be difficult to justify.

Perhaps relatively aggressive care would be acceptable if a patient had knowingly chosen that course, but we found that there had been little discussion of such a course. When we asked patients (or their families) whether they wanted CPR, 31 percent said they would rather not have it. The physicians for the patients who preferred to avoid CPR understood that preference less than half the time. Only about one-third of the patients reported any discussion with a physician about these issues, when asked in the second week of hospitalization.[16] Even when patients had written advance directives, their instructions had been discussed with a physician in only 42 percent of the cases.[17] Effective communication between patient and physician is likely to mark some very important differences in the plan of care: we found that an accord on avoiding resuscitation correlated with a reduction in hospital charges for a standard patient from $35,000 to $21,000.[18]

The problem was not just that physicians were not asking patients their views. In addition, patients were not seeking to talk with physicians about such matters as resuscitation. Of those who had not talked with a physician about CPR, only 42 percent wanted to do so.[19] Right after we asked patients their preferences concerning CPR, we asked them whether they wanted their preferences followed or would rather have their family and physicians make decisions for them. The vast majority wanted family and doctors to make the choice. Even for those who wanted no CPR and who had no family, most wanted just their doctors to make a choice later, rather than rely upon their own choice.[20]

Orders to forgo resuscitation (DNR) were often written late in the hospital stays of these patients. Although 79 percent of those who died had a DNR order by the time of death, 46 percent of these orders were written in the last two days of life.[21] Holding aside the 14 percent of DNR orders that were written on the first day of hospitalization and might reflect plans actually made in advance, 90 percent of the discussions of DNR that were documented in the chart were followed by a DNR order, usually within a day. Only 15 percent of the DNR orders written after the first three days were written for a patient who survived this hospitalization.

In other words, DNR orders were written more as last rites for a patient expected to die rather than being considered as potentially appropriate for most of the patients most of the time. This use of DNR as a marker for expected death and as a signal to change the goals of care toward symptom management and family support actually ends up working fairly well, by some measures. Unfortunately, this practice does allow for some unexpected deaths to be attended by resuscitation efforts that might well have been forgone if the possibility of a sudden death had been considered. However, the numbers are small. For most patients, a trajectory toward death was noted in time to prohibit CPR; the discussion of the issue served to give notice to the family that death was expected; and the unsettling aspects of such a discussion were avoided until death was almost certainly in store.

Only if one feels that dying should be better is the practice troubling. Not only are there some patients for whom CPR ends up being administered, but there are also many who might have wanted to be home, or to have had the chance to say good-byes, or to have been comforted for a longer time. They did not have the opportunity, because waiting until death is almost inevitable also means that most were not in any condition to talk or to transfer out of the hospital.

We also learned a great deal about the prognostication of survival time and function.[22] Building on the methods learned in APACHE II[23]— a classification system for the severity of disease—we fashioned a strategy for modeling that tested a large array of variables. Most prior models had predicted survival to some event, such as hospital discharge, and usually for a very discrete population, such as those with certain diseases being given certain treatment protocols. SUPPORT predicted the likelihood of surviving to each point in time into the next six months, drawing a curve of mortality for each patient. Our model uses sixteen measures of disease and physiology that are routinely available in hospital records. It explains about two-thirds of the variation in survival time, which is about the same as physicians' estimates. In fact, the model is improved by using the physician's estimate in addition to the sixteen physiological variables.

This model is reasonably accurate. It illuminates a number of characteristics of prognostication generally. First, prognosis for sick patients is ordinarily a deep curve, with most dying in the near future. For coma, almost 90 percent of all deaths within six months happen in the first two weeks. Even for chronic lung disease and heart failure, 50 percent of all deaths within six months are in the first month.[24] This is, in many ways, obvious since we identified patients precisely because they were hospitalized for being sick. Clearly they were at the greatest risk of death in the near future. However, it contrasts with the way people usually think, which is to assume either that there is some future time when dying is certain ("I have six months to live") or that the risks are constant over time, given that a patient has a fatal illness.

To many, it seems quite different to say that "the average person just like you will die in two weeks" and "persons like you have a 20 percent chance to live six months." Yet these are equivalent statements for persons with acute respiratory failure in SUPPORT.[25]

Even more surprising to many physicians is the degree of imprecision involved in predicting near-term death. Physicians generally think that they can tell, among hospitalized patients, who is likely to die this week, even if they know that predictions are generally not so precise. However, in SUPPORT, the median patient on the day before death had one-to-four odds of living two months. Just five days ahead of death, that median patient had a 40 percent likelihood of living two months.[26] While those are bad odds for betting, they are not hopeless and do not make pursuing treatment vigorously seem futile.

Almost everything else studied in SUPPORT varied substantially among the five sites, but prognostication did not. In other words, what treatments and diagnoses were employed, when patients and families had discussions of resuscitation, and whether patients went home quickly all differed from one site to another. However, none of these had an effect upon survival time. Once a patient this sick was in the hospital, the specifics of what was done did not seem to matter.

In addition, we were able to build a statistical model that predicts serious functional disability at two months. Its performance is nearly as good as the model for survival time.[27]

In sum, SUPPORT describes the course of a large group of persons who are dying during or after hospital care. Patients experience a great deal of vigorous medical intervention and pain, but it is not at all clear that they and their families are not agreeable to what happens. No one involved talks much—not physicians, families, or patients. Decisions are made very late in the course of the illness—a practice that risks some harm and precludes planning[28] but protects most patients from having to consider the issues at all and spares families from confronting mortality until doing so is unavoidable.

Surely we can do better. Pain could be much more of a focus. Decisions could be made in advance, and care plans shaped much more creatively. SUPPORT did try to make changes, and the intervention failed. Clearly, long-standing habits exist for myriad poorly understood reasons and do not yield readily to change. It may well be that change requires a much more fundamental restructuring of service supply, incentives, and rewards.

INSIGHTS ABOUT ENGENDERING CHANGE

SUPPORT certainly showed that it is extremely difficult to change widespread and well-integrated practices—hardly a new lesson. Nevertheless, making it easy to do things better, when physicians and others claimed that they wanted to do things better, might allow improvement. The intervention that SUPPORT started was vigorously applied and widely desired. Patients and families certainly appreciated the time with the SUPPORT nurse. Physicians were generally accepting and encouraging. But old habits turned out to be not really *that* uncomfortable, and new patterns were not really *that* much desired. Most people in such hospital settings, involved with critically ill patients, are not convinced that they are doing anything wrong. They are coping with bad situations in time-honored ways. They are comfortable with the inadequacies of present practices, even when those inadequacies are acknowledged, and they are unsettled at the prospects of new and untested patterns.

We noted that the five SUPPORT hospitals had vastly different patterns with regard to whether patients died in the hospital.[29] For a standard patient, the odds of being home to die varied almost fivefold: that patient was exceedingly likely to be at home to die in one site and exceedingly likely to die in the hospital at another. Variation this extreme was interesting, especially since we knew that the practice did not yield different survival times. We checked the usual suspects— family support, age, wealth, diagnoses, and so forth—and found no substantial explanations. Even the patient's preferences had no important impact, in part because virtually all patients want to be home if they can. We then employed the national dataset for Medicare, to determine whether this variation is found in that dataset. The SUPPORT hospitals arrayed themselves nicely over the range of Medicare regions. We then tried explaining this variation in terms of its correlation with various descriptors of the care system in those regions: bed supply, hospice utilization, nursing home supply, home care. These elements explained most of the variation in where patients die. Hospital bed supply alone is a stronger explanation than all the demographic and physiologic information put together. For every extra hospital bed per thousand Medicare beneficiaries, the chances of being in one to die went up by 5 percent. For every additional $10 per Medicare beneficiary devoted to hospices, the odds went down by almost 3 percent. These are strong effects.

The importance of these findings is not in motivating a wholesale reduction in hospital beds, though that may be warranted on other grounds. Rather, it points to the fact that what happens is what usually happens, and that patients have little opportunity, really, to shape important aspects of what happens to them. Yes, of course, a strong family with substantial resources could bring a patient home to die, even in systems that did not usually provide for that. However, patients in such systems were mostly confronted with physicians who did not follow the person at home, myriad nonstandard forms to fill

out, multiple competing service providers who do not share accountability or trust, and a system most comfortable doing exactly what it
was doing. On the other hand, persons in systems that usually got people home before death had physicians who followed the patients in all
settings, and integrated services that used the same paperwork and
people to accomplish transitions. These systems probably were comfortable living with a relative scarcity of hospital beds and had learned
to use other resources routinely.

Does that mean that it is necessarily better to die at home? No, not
at all. Persons without families, financial resources, and safe homes
almost certainly die much more miserably at home than in hospitals.
Our observation shows only that what determines whether you are likely
to die in a hospital has little to do with your preferences or disease or
financial and social status—but everything to do with the system of
social support and health care where you happen to live. If our society
decides to change the care of the dying, it almost certainly has to learn to
change important aspects of the care system and not just empower
patients with advance directives or the opportunity to communicate.

These observations are underscored in our work on advance directives. In the two years after passage of the Patient Self-Determination
Act in 1991, during Phase II, we tracked all written living wills and
durable powers of attorney, whether or not they were included in the
medical record. In short, they were ineffectual in shaping care. In fact,
the current practice of advance directive use failed at every key juncture. Despite a federal law requiring inquiry about them, only a
minority were ever documented in the record under usual conditions.
Our intervention was successful in getting virtually all advance directives recorded. However, they still had no effect upon decision making.[30] DNR orders were still considered only late in the course. People
with preferences for a DNR order and an advance directive were no
more likely to have a physician who understood than were others.
Only 12 percent of the patients had discussed the writing of an
advance directive with their physician, and they had discussed its exis-
tence with their physician only 42 percent of the time. We reviewed
all of the documents and found that 4,804 patients had written 688
documents, only 90 of which said anything specific about treatment,
and only 22 of these spoke to whether to use life-sustaining treatment
in the patient's current condition.[31]

Clearly, advance directives as they are now employed are not a considerable part of the solution. Nevertheless, the nation has invested

substantially in this approach. It is estimated to cost American hospitals up to $100 million to comply with the Patient Self-Determination Act.[32] Many voluntary public organizations, lawyers, ethicists, and professional organizations have promoted advance directives. The rates of use have increased, but their actual effectiveness seems disappointingly small. Perhaps this is because the advance directives were not enough to disrupt the strong effects of habits and usual practices. Patients who have such directives are perhaps lulled into thinking that they have done something important and have solved their personal risks of overtreatment. Yet even when a patient has such a directive, care systems are allowed to continue on their usual course, not even having to undertake effective communication about the intent of the patient in writing the directive. A cynic might say that the work to promote advance directives is proving to be a lot of "sound and fury, signifying nothing," and that the work was acceptable to doctors and hospitals precisely because the directives mean little.

Other forms of advance directives, or these forms in other populations, or improved practices of advance care planning that are not so tightly linked to legal forms might well be much more effective. We would look to build upon SUPPORT's finding that for almost all of these very sick patients there was a time at or just before admission to the hospital when they were capable of making plans.[33] Further innovation and evaluation is urgently needed in order to guide policy and practice. We now feel that medical practice should incorporate progressive and pervasive advance care planning appropriate to the patient's clinical situation, and especially aiming at planning the response to predictable serious complications.[34] This proposal should be implemented and evaluated, as should other appealing proposals for improvement.

INSIGHTS ABOUT THE POWER OF MYTHS

John F. Kennedy once said, "The great enemy of the truth is very often not the lie—deliberate, contrived, and dishonest—but the myth—persistent, persuasive, and unrealistic."[35] How true. Some things are so widely believed that our data were taken as confirming them, even when our conclusions were quite different. When the main findings about the intervention were released, in November 1995, headlines included these: "American Way of Dying Examined: Doctors Ignorant of Patients' Wishes, New Study Reveals"; "U.S. Hospitals' Way of Death

Resists Change: Study Finds Care Depersonalized, Impervious to Patients' Wishes"; and "Dying Patients' Wishes Often Ignored: Study says Doctors, Hospitals Prolong Agony, Expense." This is not what we said and not what our press release said. We stated, correctly, that patients had preferences that were not understood by physicians, and that neither patients nor physicians were talking about them. Nevertheless, we spent a great deal of time in the ensuing days trying to talk reporters out of scapegoating physicians. They clearly wanted to write about arrogant doctors and pleading patients. Imagine our surprise when we found that the headline in the press release issued by the *Journal of the American Medical Association*, which we had not seen before, said, "Care for Dying Americans Needs Substantial Improvement, Say Researchers in Largest-Ever Study of People Near Death: Study Finds Too Many Die Alone, in Pain, and Attached to Machines." Even the public relations people for physicians seemed to point the blame at doctors.

As we worked with the press, over and over we explained that the problem was much more difficult than that doctors did not hear their patients' requests; it was that no one involved was talking about these subjects. This was clearly not as good a story, and it was often not written. What showed up was the mistaken notion that patients could not get a hearing.

Similarly, the public assumes that we are spending too much money on dying people and that such outlays should be easy to stop. I appeared on a number of call-in radio shows, and someone would invariably call in to say that she had these problems all solved for herself because she had a living will. I would ask what it said, and the response would be that "treatment should stop when it becomes clear that I will die." When the caller was asked to clarify her wishes about treatment, she replied that treatment would stop when the situation was "hopeless." When I asked *how* hopeless the situation would have to be, or how close death had to be, the caller would predictably become testy—saying that this would be obvious. Then the caller or the host would note that doctors were just greedy and stupid in throwing lots of treatment at conditions where it was obviously futile. Often, I think I managed to force some openness by giving the data about how uncertain death is, right up to a time near its occurrence. People seemed stunned to learn that for the average person in SUPPORT the odds of living for another two months were fifty-fifty *just a week* ahead of death. However, it was very difficult to have them translate this into a recognition that the resources spent do not seem wasted until *after* the death. Before the death, they seem more like vigorous efforts to help a struggling person pull through. Afterward, they come to seem like a waste. The public must believe that physicians are quite prescient in order to think that treatment can be withheld from only the right patients.

The notion that we might save lots of money and suffering just by banning "futile" care has been enjoying widespread currency; it was dealt a major blow by SUPPORT. We simulated the effect of a policy to ban life-sustaining medical treatment for persons who had, on their third study day, a prognosis of less than 1 percent to live for two months.[36] At the 1 percent level, 115 people (out of 4,301 in Phase I SUPPORT) would have had treatment stopped, saving about 10 percent of their hospital expenditures. One-third of the patients did have a ventilator withdrawn, expecting death, and 83 died within two days. Three-quarters of the potential savings would rely upon just 12 patients, most of whom were young and with good functional status, and half of whom were trying to recover from a transplant. This work makes it clear that a "rule" that barred life-sustaining treatment from being used when the chances of survival were small would have little impact and would be very hard to apply.

While SUPPORT illuminated the difficulties of finding easy solutions to costs and suffering, it also underscored the devastating impact of these serious illnesses on families. We found that one-third of families lost all or most of their savings, and that more than half had at least one major disruption in living arrangements, employment, schooling, or other plans. Families endured these serious problems despite the fact that 96 percent of SUPPORT patients had health insurance.[37] We have recently shown that families facing these overwhelming burdens are more likely to feel that the patient prefers comfort care rather than aggressive care.[38]

SUPPORT headlines trumpeted our findings on pain and dying on ventilators, and that is important. However, SUPPORT did not really collect information on the inner life experience of patients and families. This sort of information is not part of cultural myth, research studies, or popular stories. My experience in hospice care showed me that dying people and those around them can often grow greatly in understanding, can enhance relationships, and can do important personal work in their last weeks. Yet the fact that dying can grant meaning to life—the patient's and the family's—is not part of our cultural understanding. Instead, dying is just awful. Dying better is perceived to be merely less awful.

Americans also endorse a language and a conceptualization of the course of serious disease as entailing, at some point, a "transition from cure to care," finding no comfort in middling pathways. The care plan has to be conceived as aiming at cure or accepting of death, with very little time spent in transition. This is curious. For most of the diseases we studied, there is no cure, and there has not been since the time of diagnosis. What self-deception allows us to talk of cardiac medications or respirators as curative? Furthermore, people want "caring" through-out. We certainly would rather not suffer unnecessarily, even in the context of pursuing substantial prolongations of life span. Yet the idea that Americans want many things from medicine and that their pri-oritization admits of many possibilities is not popular. Instead, peo-ple ritualize the mantra of "transition from cure to care."

In SUPPORT, interestingly, there were mostly periods of a "full court press" until a transition to "comfort care." Very few care plans pursued ventilators and DNR orders simultaneously, for example. Instead, the DNR followed on the incipient failure of the ICU.

Medical care actually has many goals: preventing disease and dis-ability, rehabilitating, prolonging life, curing disease, maintaining function, explaining and predicting change, restoring control, and eas-ing suffering, for example. Ordinarily, people want them all; but in most circumstances, not all can be achieved, and in some circum-stances achieving some goals entails limiting the attainment of oth-ers. Devising a plan of care requires acknowledging which goals might be achieved and being thoughtful over time about the merits of vari-ous approaches over time.

Perhaps our eagerness to have a transition from cure to care reflects our eagerness to be "other than dying" most of the time. As long as we claim to be pursuing cure, we are to be counted among the "living"—a group I sometimes label "the temporarily immortal." Once we have to accept that there is no cure but only caring, then we must acknowl-edge our impending mortality, and we join the "dying." While it is an acceptable cultural compromise for each of us to be counted among the "dying" for a period at the end of life, we want that period to be short, unavoidable, and closely tied to actual death. We do not want to be "dying" for years, or through multiple cycles of serious illness and substantial recovery. Thus, having an illusion of pursuing cure as long as the claim is not seen as silly, and of transitioning to pursuing "care" when death is close upon us, may be a way to keep from having to deal with death most of our lives. The American culture finds that appealing.

The timing of DNR orders in SUPPORT shows the effect of such a structuring of reality. Most were written as prognoses for survival dropped and within a few days of actual death. Mostly, there had not been explicit discussions with patients or families about how to plan for the likelihood of death until this discussion was undertaken. Until then, patients and families "knew" that the illness was serious, but they still thought they could beat the odds. One patient told us, "My doctor says I have 20 percent chance to live six months, but I know that I will be in that 20 percent." Another husband told his wife, "That's 25 percent, honey, that's just one of these four fingers, grab it, grab it." They were generally so optimistic about their prospects that those who acknowledged having a prognosis of 90 percent or less to live two months were dramatically more likely to prefer DNR orders and to want to talk with physicians about plans.[39] It was as if one could talk about rescue only until it was out of reach. Then one could talk about dying, but at that point it was often too late to change the care plan much.

The way we structure our experience—the framing we impose and the language we use—delimits what is possible. If we strongly believe, wrongly, that it is just the blindness and deafness of physicians that gets in the way of good care, we mistakenly intervene in their education and practice rather than addressing our shared responsibilities. If we structure the course of fatal illness to have a long period of pursuit of cure, followed by a short period of dying, we fail to seek out the full possibilities for worthy living throughout the course. SUPPORT's intervention may well have failed to have an effect in large part because it accepted the conventional cultural understandings rather than challenging or changing them.

INSIGHTS ON DECISION MAKING

Public language describes virtually all history in terms of choices and decisions. We say that "it was decided to use a ventilator," or "My doctor chose to put me in the hospital because I was breathing so hard." In medical ethics and law, virtually all actions are spoken of as decisions, and statements of optimum care systems focus heavily on optimum decision making. In a trivial sense, of course, such language is not inaccurate. For almost any action, another action was possible, and could have been "chosen." It is not at all clear, however, that the putative decision maker sees the options in this way.

An artist puts a daub of orange paint on a canvas in a certain way. We would not usually say he had "chosen" to paint that way. We would probably focus upon his overall vision and intent. He created that sunset with certain methods and paints. It is satisfying or not, in various ways, and we can critique his method, his vision, or his result. However, we are not likely to do so in terms of his "decisions." In much the same way, creating a life may seem more like painting, and less like a decision tree, than we usually acknowledge. We follow some pathways because they are well-trod, or because they appeal to our sense of who we are, or for emotional reasons, rather than their being justified by having the highest expected yield of benefit compared with other possibilities. We may never actually have held the other possibilities in mind.

Furthermore, what often really shapes the patient's experience might well not have been a real decision at all. Consider how often patients and families say, quite naturally, "The doctor decided that Mary needed to go to the hospital." For a person who may be dying, that is one of the most significant decisions to be made, yet it is not common in many settings for it to be posed to anyone. On the other hand, decisions about resuscitation are posed for virtually all patients, yet they actually make little difference. The patient for whom we are willing to weigh the merits of resuscitation is almost certain to be sick enough not to survive a resuscitation attempt. Furthermore, these issues will keep being raised until the care team gets permission for a DNR order, so the family that "decides" to have CPR today is likely to be convinced to see things differently tomorrow. Such a "choice" reflects a frail sense of self-determination.

SUPPORT patients and families often seemed adrift, confused, and in need of guidance about what was happening and how to respond to it. Intervention nurses spent a great deal of time explaining how a hospital works, the nature of the illness, and the resources available to help. Often, patients or family members would claim that he or she "needs to know what to do now." In a conceptual framework that assumes that decisions are what counts, they would have been understood to be seeking well-constructed decision trees and ways to elicit preferences. Taken at their word, however, they may really have simply been seeking "a way to proceed." Especially since their "choice" will be ratified by their physician, patients and families may well want "a way to proceed" more than they want to have spent a lot of effort and anxiety in seeking for a "slightly better way to proceed." When one makes choices, one bears the responsibility for them. One way to avoid some of the regret that follows when things don't work out well is to be sure that the course taken is "what most people would do," which may well be what was being sought in asking "how to proceed."

If these notions are true, then it is curious that we express ourselves in terms of decisions and decision making. What would be the alternative? We could simply say that thus and so was what happened, but then we sound so irrelevant. We could say that we followed the usual pathway for such situations, but that is no more satisfying. In short, we seem to like the illusion of being in control. Furthermore, as mentioned above, the discussion of DNR might signal a more important transition to acknowledging the likely immanence of death, so some of our "decisions" may function as important rituals rather than as real choices.

In any case, with whatever language, if "decisions" for the very sick merely reflect patterned behavior more often than they reflect what the patient and the family want, then reform need not start with improved information and the enabling of better decisions. It might be much better to reshape the incentives that create and sustain the patterns. In other words, reform could start with a reduction in the number of hospital beds and an increase in home care, or valuing physicians' skills in pain control or communication rather than in adjusting cardiac output.

INSIGHTS ABOUT THE MERITS OF MEDICAL INTERVENTIONS

SUPPORT thus far has done three evaluations of the merits of medical interventions in this population, and all three give less-than-robust encouragement to the enthusiasts of medical treatment. First, we assessed the population rate of SUPPORT-like illnesses in the Marshfield, Wisconsin area.[40] Some had thought that it would be uncommon to survive very long without vigorous treatment for such serious illnesses. Instead, we found that, for respiratory failure, more than half of the patients with illness severe enough to qualify were not coming into the study. Those not enrolled were generally older persons, often disabled with chronic disease, and often in nursing homes. Some never came to the hospital, and some who did were treated in regular wards, not in the intensive care unit. Whereas one-third of those who received ICU care and were enrolled in SUPPORT did die, two-thirds of those not enrolled died. Their worse baseline status undoubtedly explains some of that, and surely there is some merit to the vigorous treatment that pulled others through in intensive care. However, this comparison shows that it is not the case that all who do not get that care die. It is an error of hubris to claim that forgoing intubation, ventilation, close monitoring, and aggressive care is tantamount to certain death.

The doubt about therapeutic optimism that arises here is buttressed by the observation that substantial site variations in all measured aspects of practice were not reflected in differences in survival time. This makes it likely that one could theoretically reduce each intervention, including communication, to the lowest level found at any site and not affect survival time overall. It is an interesting and humbling possibility.

The most striking finding in SUPPORT to date concerning the merits of our usual interventions is a study of the effects of right heart catheterization.[41] We had a large number of patients (5,735) who had conditions sometimes managed with right heart catheterization—a procedure that involves placing a special intravenous line into the heart and measuring pressures there. We were able to develop a scoring system that predicted the likelihood of having a right heart cath. Within each 10 percent of likelihood, some had the procedure and some did not. If right heart catheterization were a benefit, then those who got it should do somewhat better than expected in terms of survival, and those who did not should do somewhat less well. That was not what happened. In every stratum, having a cath was associated with slightly *less* good survival. In fact, in each disease type and site, the same association holds. In other words, there was no population for whom the procedure seemed to confer a benefit.

Of course, our findings will have to be confirmed elsewhere, and there are shortcomings to our study design, but the doubt these data raise should be powerful in motivating valid assessments of the merits of continuing to use right heart cath in these sick patients. It is done about 1.7 million times each year, at a direct cost of about $2,000 each time and carrying associated costs of more than $8,000, for a total of $17 billion a year.

If the effect of right heart cath is harmful in this way, only a study this large and complex could show it. Not only is this finding important for its call to study the merits of this particular widely used procedure, but it is also important for illuminating an approach to evaluating a number of other procedures that have not been well assessed before being put into widespread use.

CONCLUSIONS

SUPPORT was a remarkable undertaking, achieved by the collaborative efforts of hundreds of people who were bound together by caring to learn how to improve the experience of seriously ill people. Data quality was high, interviewees felt well treated, and the institutions were most cooperative.

SUPPORT is teaching us a great deal. Some of what we learned was expected. We learned to make better prognostic models, predict function as well as survival time, and describe outcomes and decision-making practices.

SUPPORT also turned out to be the largest study of dying ever done in America. The insights about how we approach dying and what patients and families experience will undoubtedly serve to anchor understanding for some time.

SUPPORT also is yielding some unexpected insights: the nature of change and agents of change, the role of decisions, the merits of treatments. It is a first look at an important field. There is much to learn before we fully understand serious illness and death and how to serve people facing them.

Endnotes

1. The President's Commission for the Study of Ethical Problems in Medicine and Biomedical and Behavioral Research, *Deciding to Forego Life Sustaining Treatment*, (Washington, D.C.: U.S. Govt. Printing Office, 1983).

2. D. J. Murphy and L. E. Cluff, "Introduction: The SUPPORT Study," *J Clin Epidemiol* 43 Suppl. (1990), v–viii; J. Lynn, J. Johnson, and R. J. Levine, "The Ethical Conduct of Health Services Research: A Case Study of 55 Institutions' Applications to the SUPPORT Project," *Clin Res* 42 (1994), 3–10.

    The ICU Research Unit at the George Washington University Medical Center was the National Coordinating Center (NCC) for this study, codirected by William Knaus and Joanne Lynn. Lynn was at the Center for the Evaluative Clinical Sciences at Dartmouth College for 1992–1995 and then director of the Center to Improve Care of the Dying at the George Washington University. Knaus moved to chair the new Department of Health Evaluation Sciences at the University of Virginia in 1995. The five hospitals and their lead investigators were (1) Beth Israel Hospital in Boston, Lee Goldman (now at University of California at San Francisco) and Russell S. Phillips; (2) Cleveland MetroHealth Medical Center, Alfred F. Connors, Jr., and Neal V. Dawson; (3) Duke University Medical Center, William J. Fulkerson; (4) Marshfield Medical Research Foundation, Norman A. Desbiens, Peter Layde (now at the Medical College of Wisconsin) and Steven Broste; and (5) UCLA School of Medicine, Robert K. Oye and Neil Wenger. Frank Harrell (now at the University of Virginia) led the study's national Statistical Center at Duke University. Marilyn Bergner (deceased) and Albert Wu from The Johns Hopkins University were involved in the National Coordinating Center. The study depended upon the contributions of dozens of additional investigators, study supervisors, record abstractors, interviewers, intervention nurses, and data managers.

3. D. J. Murphy and L.E. Cluff, eds., "The SUPPORT Study." *J Clin Epidemiol* 43 Suppl. (1990), 11S–28S; W. A. Knaus, F. E. Harrell, J. Lynn, L. Goldman, R. S. Phillips, A. F. Connors, N. V. Dawson, W. J. Fulkerson, R. M. Califf, N. Desbiens, P. Layde, R. K. Oye, P. E. Bellamy, R. B. Hakim, and D. P. Wagner, "The SUPPORT Prognostic Model: Objective Estimates of Survival for Seriously Ill Hospitalized Adults," *Ann Intern Med* 122 (1995), 191–203.

4. Knaus and others (1995).

5. A. W. Wu, A. M. Damiano, J. Lynn, C. Alzola, J. Teno, C. S. Landefeld, N. Desbiens, J. Tsevat, A. Mayer-Oakes, F. E. Harrell, Jr., and W. A. Knaus, "Predicting Future Functional Status for Seriously Ill Hospitalized Adults: the SUPPORT Prognostic Model," *Ann Intern Med* 122 (1995), 342–350.

6. SUPPORT Principal Investigators, "A Controlled Trial to Improve Care for Seriously Ill Hospitalized Patients: The Study to Understand Prognoses and Preferences for Outcomes and Risks of Treatments (SUPPORT)," *JAMA* 274 (1995), 1591–1598.

7. SUPPORT Principal Investigators (1995).

8. P. M. Layde, S. K. Broste, N. Desbiens, M. Follen, J. Lynn, D. Reding, and H. Vidaillet, "Generalizability of Clinical Studies Conducted at Tertiary Care Medical Centers: A Population-Based Analysis," *J Clin Epidemiol* 49 (1996), 835–841.

9. SUPPORT Principal Investigators (1995).

10. SUPPORT Principal Investigators (1995).

11. SUPPORT Principal Investigators (1995).

12. J. Lynn, J. M. Teno, R. S. Phillips, A. W. Wu, N. Desbiens, J. Harrold, M. T. Claessens, N. Wenger, B. Kreling, and A. F. Connors, Jr., for the SUPPORT Investigators, "Perceptions by Family Members of the Dying Experience of Older and Seriously Ill Patients," *Annals of Internal Medicine* 126 (1997), 97–106.

13. SUPPORT Principal Investigators (1995).

14. J. A. Patterson, J. M. Teno, J. Lynn, and others for the SUPPORT Investigators, "Who Gets CPR as They Die? Variation by Disease, Race, and Hospital," *J Am Geriat Soc* 43 (1995), SA54.

15. Lynn and others (1997).

16. SUPPORT Principal Investigators (1995).

17. J. Teno, J. Lynn, N. Wenger, R. Phillips, D. Murphy, A. F. Connors, Jr., N. Desbiens, W. Fulkerson, P. Bellamy, and W. Knaus, "Advance Directives for Seriously Ill Hospitalized Patients: Effectiveness with the Patient Self-Determination Act and the SUPPORT intervention," *J. Am. Geriat. Soc.* (forthcoming).

18. J. M. Teno, R. B. Hakim, W. A. Knaus, N. S. Wenger, R. S. Phillips, A. W. Wu, P. Layde, A. F. Connors, Jr., N. V. Dawson, and J. Lynn for the SUPPORT Investigators, "Preferences for Cardiopulmonary Resuscitation: Physician-Patient Agreement and Hospital Resource Use," *J Gen Intern Med* 10 (1995), 179–186.

19. J. C. Hofmann, N. S. Wenger, R. B. Davis, J. Teno, A. F. Connors, N. Desbiens, J. Lynn, and R. S. Phillips for the SUPPORT Investigators, "Patients' Preferences for Communication with Physicians About End-of-Life Decisions," *Annals Int Med* (forthcoming).

20. J. Lynn, J. Teno, R. S. Phillips, R. E. Phillips, N. Wenger, B. Virnig, A. Connors, and A. Galanos for the HELP Investigators, "Preferences for Instructional Directives or Family Decision Making Among Older Patients," *J Am Geriatr Soc* 42 (1994), 217.

21. SUPPORT Principal Investigators (1995).

22. Knaus and others (1995); Wu and others (1995); F. E. Harrell, Jr., K. L. Lee, and D. B. Mark, "Tutorial in Biostatistics: Multivariable Prognostic Models: Issues in Developing Models, Evaluating Assumptions and Adequacy, and Measuring and Reducing Errors," *Statistics in Medicine* 15 (1996), 361–387; J. Lynn, J. M. Teno, and F. E. Harrell, Jr., "Accurate Prognostications of Death: Opportunities and Challenges for Clinicians. Caring for Patients at the End of Life [Special Issue]," *West J Med* 163 (1995), 250–257.

23. W. A. Knaus, E. A. Draper, D. P. Wagner, and J. E. Zimmerman, "APACHE II: A Severity of Disease Classification System," *Crit Care Med* 13 (1985), 818–829.

24. Knaus and others (1995).

25. Lynn, Teno, and Harrell (1995).

26. J. Lynn, F. E. Harrell, Jr., and F. Cohn, "Defining the 'Terminally Ill': Insights from SUPPORT," *Duquesne L. Rev.* 35 (1996), 311–336; F. Harrell, Jr., F. Cohn, D. Wagner, and A. F. Connors, Jr., "Prognosis of Seriously Ill Hospitalized Patients on the Days Before Death: Implications for Patient Care and Public Policy," *New Horizons* 5 (1997), 55–61.

27. Wu and others (1995).

28. N. S. Wenger, R. K. Oye, P. E. Bellamy, J. Lynn, R. S. Phillips, N. A. Desbiens, P. Kussin, and S. J. Younger for the SUPPORT Investigators, "Prior Capacity of Patients Lacking Decision Making Ability Early in Hospitalization," *J Gen Intern Med* 9 (1994), 539–543.

29. R. Pritchard, J. Teno, E. Fisher, and others, for the SUPPORT Investigators, "Regional Variation in the Place of Death," *J Gen Intern Med* 9 (1994), 146A.

30. J. M. Teno, S. Licks, J. Lynn, N. Wenger, A. F. Connors, R. Phillips, M. A. O'Connor, D. Murphy, W. J. Fulkerson, N. Desbiens, and W. Knaus for the SUPPORT Investigators, "Do Advanced Directives Provide Instructions Which Direct Care?" *J. Am. Geriat. Soc.* 45 (1997), 508–512; J. Teno, J. Lynn, A. F. Connors, N. Wenger, R. S. Phillips, C. Alzola, D. Murphy, N. Desbiens, and W. A. Knaus for the SUPPORT Investigators, "The Illusion of End of Life Resource Savings with Advance Directives," *J. Am. Geriat. Soc.* 45 (1997) 513–518; J. M. Teno, J. Lynn, R. S. Phillips, D. Murphy, S. J. Youngner, P. Bellamy, A. F. Connors, Jr., N. A. Desbiens, W. Fulkerson, and W. A. Knaus, "Do Formal Advanced Directives Affect Resuscitation Decisions and the Use of Resources for Seriously Ill Patients?" *J Clin Ethics* 5 (1994), 23–30.

31. Teno, Licks, and others (1997).

32. J. Sugarman, N. R. Powe, D. A. Brillantes, and M. K. Smith, "The Cost of Ethics Legislation: A Look at the Patient Self-Determination Act," *Kennedy Institute of Ethics Journal* 3 (1993), 387–399.

33. Wenger and others (1994).

34. J. M. Teno and J. Lynn, "Putting Advance Care Planning into Action," *Journal of Clinical Ethics* 7 (1996), 205–213.

35. L. L. Levinson, *Bartlett's Unfamiliar Quotations* (Chicago: Cowles, 1971) p. 17.

36. J. Teno, D. Murphy, J. Lynn, A. Tosteson, N. Desbiens, A. F. Connors, Jr., M. B. Hamel, A. Wu, R. Phillips, N. Wenger, F. E. Harrell, Jr., and W. Knaus,

"Prognosis-Based Futility Guidelines: Does Anyone Win? *J. Am. Geriat. Soc.* 42 (1994), 1202–1207.

37. K. E. Covinsky, L. Goldman, E. F. Cook, R. Oye, N. Desbiens, D. Reding, W. Fulkerson, A. F. Connors, J. Lynn, and R. S. Phillips for the SUPPORT Investigators, "The Impact of Serious Illness on Patients' Families," *JAMA* 272 (1994), 1839–1844.

38. K. E. Covinsky, S. Landefeld, J. Teno, A. F. Connors, N. Dawson, S. Youngner, N. Desbiens, J. Lynn, W. Fulkerson, D. Reding, R. Oye, and R. S. Phillips for the SUPPORT Investigators, "Is Economic Hardship on the Families of the Seriously Ill Associated with Patient and Surrogate Care Preferences?" *Arch Intern Med* 156 (1996), 1737–1741.

39. S. J. O'Day, J. C. Weeks, E. F. Cook, L. M. Peterson, N. Wenger, D. Reding, F. E. Harrell, W. Fulkerson, N. V. Dawson, A. Connors, W. Knaus, and R. S. Phillips, and the SUPPORT Investigators, "Relationship Between Cancer Patients, Predictions of Prognosis, and Their Treatment Preferences," *Clin Res* 41 (1993), 579a.

40. Layde and others (1996).

41. A. F. Connors, T. Speroff, N. V. Dawson, C. Thomas, F. E. Harrell, Jr., D. Wagner, N. Desbiens, L. Goldman, A. W. Wu, R. M. Califf, W. J. Fulkerson, Jr., H. Vidaillet, S. Broste, P. Bellamy, J. Lynn, and W. A. Knaus for the SUPPORT Investigators, "The Effectiveness of Right Heart Catheterization in the Initial Care of Critically Ill Patients," *JAMA* 276 (1996), 889–897.

‑‑‑ Developing Child Immunization Registries

The All Kids Count Program

Gordon H. DeFriese
Kathleen M. Faherty
Victoria A. Freeman
Priscilla A. Guild
Delores A. Musselman
William C. Watson, Jr.
Kristin Nicholson Saarlas

Editors' Introduction

Many of the social problems affecting the health of Americans do not have known technical solutions. As a society, we continue to struggle with questions about how to convince people to stop smoking or to be less violent, how to improve the way health care services are coordinated for people with Alzheimer's or how to finance such services equitably. But in the area of early childhood diseases—such as measles and whooping cough—we have well-known technical solutions for reducing the incidence of these diseases. Available vaccines can dramatically reduce the onset of a wide range of childhood diseases, and the vaccines are not particularly expensive or difficult to administer.

So the goal of immunizing all or most children should be attainable. As a nation, however, we have not succeeded at getting some children from low-income families—and particularly younger children—vaccinated. Barriers to medical care generally facing these families lead to low vaccination rates.

Chapter Nine reviews a national program supported by the Foundation and other funders to use computer technology to design vaccination registries that facilitate the monitoring of childhood immunizations and allow outreach workers to get in touch with the families of children needing vaccinations. The program supported a range of efforts in twenty-four geographic areas to improve immunization rates for very young children.

As this chapter makes clear, even when technical solutions to a social problem exist, there are incredibly complex issues of implementation that need to be addressed. It explains in detail the barriers faced and some of the creative solutions devised by many of the grantees to make these registry systems work. The chapter also sets the work of the grantees into a context of the problems associated with immunization in this country.

This chapter is a collaboration between a team of researchers at the University of North Carolina and the national program office based at the Carter Presidential Center in Atlanta. The lead author is Gordon H. DeFriese, director and professor of social medicine, epidemiology, and health policy and administration at the Cecil G. Sheps Center for Health Services Research of the University of North Carolina at Chapel Hill. DeFriese led the team that conducted the national evaluation of All Kids Count for the Foundation. Kathleen M. Faherty coordinated the center's efforts in evaluating the Foundation's national All Kids Count project. Victoria A. Freeman is a research associate at the Sheps Center. Priscilla A. Guild is deputy director for administrative operations at the Sheps Center and a co-investigator on the evaluation of All Kids Count. Delores A. Musselman is a social research assistant at the Sheps Center. William C. Watson, Jr., is deputy director for the All Kids Count project and was director of operations for the Carter Presidential Center. Kristin Nicholson Saarlas is the assistant deputy director of All Kids Count.

The United States has achieved the highest immunization levels for preschool children ever recorded, but we still may not be doing enough to protect them from diseases that can be prevented by vaccination. As impressive as the rates are, a quarter of the nation's very young children have still not completed their basic immunization series on time. The societal consequences of this lapse were directly illustrated in the late 1980s, when an epidemic of fifty thousand cases of measles resulted in some eleven thousand hospitalizations and the death of 130 children nationwide.[1] Such problems motivated The Robert Wood Johnson Foundation to launch the national All Kids Count childhood immunization initiative in 1991. This program sought to identify communities and states that were capable of developing immunization monitoring and follow-up systems to "improve and sustain access to immunizations for preschool children."

The rate of immunization is very high for children who are old enough to enter school—as high as 95 percent, including all recommended vaccines in most jurisdictions—but this level has been achieved only through public health laws that require proof of immunizations before the students enroll. For preschool age children, the rates have been much lower—reaching an all-time high of 75 percent in 1995. Fortunately, the incidence of vaccine-preventable diseases has dropped sharply; in 1995 it was at the lowest reported level ever. The number of measles cases reported nationwide was below three hundred, compared to twenty-seven thousand cases in 1990.[2]

Despite this evidence of progress, however, estimates derived from the National Immunization Survey by the Centers for Disease Control and Prevention's National Immunization Program (CDC/NIP) indicated that in 1995 approximately 25 percent of preschool-age children had not received at least one dose of the recommended series of vaccines.[3] The failure to meet the minimum levels of immunization for preschool-age children—90 percent coverage for measles; diphtheria and tetanus toxoids and pertussis (DTP); polio; and *Haemophilus influenzae* type b (Hib); and 70 percent coverage for hepatitis B—is cause for serious concern.[4] Such failures impose not only a public health risk but also financial costs that are associated with diagnosing and treating the illnesses. It is estimated that every dollar spent on MMR® vaccine can result in a saving of twenty-one dollars in future medical care costs.[5]

The National Immunization Program of the CDC aimed at increasing immunization levels so that:

- By 1996, at least 90 percent of children under the age of two would have received the initial and most critical doses of the recommended vaccine series.

- By the year 2000, at least 90 percent of the children under age two will have received the complete series of routinely recommended vaccines.

- By the year 2000 and beyond, a sustainable system will be established that ensures a level of 90 percent coverage of all two-year-old children with all recommended vaccines.

Although the nation appears to be well on its way to meeting these goals, a gap of 15 percentage points remains between the national goal of 90 percent coverage for the year 2000 and the 1995 average of 75 percent for children age 19–35 months. Once that gap is closed, however, perhaps the most daunting challenge facing us is that of *sustaining* levels of 90 percent coverage, once attained, into the next century.

The potential consequences of this unmet public health need are clear, but there nonetheless continue to be many barriers to immunization for preschool children. Most children in this country receive all the medical care they need from single health-care providers, yet many poor children lack a regular source of primary medical care, and many low-income parents must rely on hospital emergency rooms to deal with the medical needs of their children.[6] Many health insurance plans available to families do not cover the costs of childhood immunizations, and there is considerable variability among state Medicaid programs in the extent of coverage for these services, leaving these as out-of-pocket costs to be borne by parents.[7]

When we take these many barriers and systemic problems into account, it is evident that economic considerations are only one of the many reasons for the underimmunization of preschool children. Even when the vaccines are made free for children whose parents cannot pay, as happened after the passage of the Comprehensive Childhood Immunization Act of 1993 and establishment of its Vaccines for Children Program, inadequate immunization rates persisted in many areas. Besides the problem of ensuring adequate insurance coverage and access to regular pediatric care for all children, child health care providers have often found it difficult to determine which preschool patients who come to them for other reasons actually need immunizations.[8]

Many providers miss opportunities to immunize young children who are brought to them for care by not checking the child's immunization status at the time of these visits or because the records are incomplete. This may be because the child is a new patient or has been taken to several providers. Add to this the relatively complicated—at least in the minds of some parents—nature of the recommended immunization series and the fairly mobile nature of many American families, and the barriers to full early childhood immunization coverage continue to be significant.

These barriers must be taken into account when considering the potential for *sustaining* the higher rates of immunization coverage that have already been achieved and to which we still aspire, since these rates were achieved at great expense, in terms of money, time, and effort contributed by public and private organizations. These have involved the extensive efforts of private companies and many dedicated civic organizations in communities nationwide in bringing about multimedia public awareness campaigns, incentives to parents to immunize their children, door-to-door campaigns, and immunization opportunities in countless shopping malls and health fairs. President and Mrs. Clinton have directed considerable attention to these efforts, as have elected and appointed officials at all levels; the CDC; and a host of federal, state, and local agencies. To what extent can we expect these efforts to continue year after year? What will it take to achieve and maintain our goal of realizing the public health potential of the vaccines at our disposal?

Informed observers of this situation argue for multiple interventions structured to meet the needs of different regions and populations. Among the strategies most often discussed, one stands out as meriting special attention: the establishment of comprehensive, computer-based information systems, at the state or local level, to monitor the immunization status of individual children and trigger efforts to assist children who are not being immunized. For these systems to deal with the entire population of preschool children in a community, they should be accessible to, and involve the participation of, all immunization providers. Then they should be used to facilitate service delivery through coordinated outreach and follow-up measures. Finally, the systems should be used to determine coverage rates for individual and institutional providers and to target populations in need of more attention. (Although the National Immunization Survey provides annual immunization coverage data for states and municipalities, there is some concern that the survey methodology does not permit the identification of smaller areas or populations that are seriously underimmunized.[9])

THE ROBERT WOOD JOHNSON FOUNDATION'S RESPONSE

Although the CDC had piloted automatic immunization registry systems in eleven state and local health departments between 1979 and 1985, there was no organized extension of this concept until the measles outbreaks in the early 1990s called attention to low immunization coverage levels. In 1991, motivated by these problems and their potential solutions, the Foundation launched the All Kids Count Childhood Immunization Initiative. It stated in its solicitation of proposals:

> The purpose of this initiative, called All Kids Count, is to establish immunization monitoring and follow-up systems that—when combined with other local, state, and federal immunization efforts—will help increase immunization rates among preschool children and reduce rates of illness, disability, and death from vaccine-preventable diseases.[10]

The Foundation sought to identify communities and states that were capable of developing these immunization monitoring and follow-up systems. In 1991, there were few local or statewide immunization registry systems that were fully operational and included the full participation of both public- and private-sector providers. The effort by the Foundation had the support of the CDC, which was preparing to stimulate state registry planning efforts.

Although these ideas had been discussed before 1991, when All Kids Count was launched, no consensus existed regarding the technology that should be used to support these registry systems, and the cost of starting and maintaining the systems was relatively unknown. Consequently, applicants for All Kids Count planning grants were allowed considerable latitude in the direction their efforts would take, in the shape and scope of the immunization registries they would develop, and in the way these efforts would unfold.

The Foundation received 114 proposals, and in November 1992 twenty-three applicants were given one-year planning grants of up to $150,000. In November 1993, fourteen of these projects received grants from the Foundation, in most cases for two years, to launch their efforts. Twelve of the projects have received an additional two years' funding, for a possible total of $525,000 per project over four years.

The family of All Kids Count initiative projects was expanded significantly when four additional projects were supported by the Packard Foundation, two additional projects were assisted by the Annie E. Casey Foundation, and three more were funded (one each) by the California Wellness Foundation, the Flinn Foundation, and the Skillman Foundation. In addition, The Robert Wood Johnson Foundation made a special grant to fund a statewide childhood immunization effort in New Jersey in 1993. This brought the total of All Kids Count projects to twenty-four, including six statewide and eighteen municipal or county-based projects. Most of the All Kids Count grantees are based in public health department immunization units that also receive support from the CDC.

ISSUES AND CONSIDERATIONS IN NATIONAL PROGRAM DEVELOPMENT

The All Kids Count initiative illustrates how an idea that is simple in concept can be complex and difficult in practice. The technology and protocols needed to develop registries may be routine in fields like law enforcement and motor vehicle registration, but they are not so easy in the field of public health. The task is complicated by the American system being built around a loose (and often ineffective) intersection of public- and private-sector responsibilities for child health care. These sectors must cooperate in the process of monitoring a series of immunizations for each child over a period of at least two years, during which child and family names, child guardianship, and residences may change. The great data management and technological challenges are compounded by the numerous providers using, entering, and accessing the systems. Also, some groups are suspicious of computerized monitoring of individuals, even for a good cause, and have occasionally objected to immunization registries as invasion of privacy.

This tension between the public good and the individual rights of citizens is being played out in other, more publicized and generally more controversial arenas; it may continue to be an issue as the registries reach full operation and if (or when) data linkages are instituted between registries.

Defining Immunization Registry Systems

When The Robert Wood Johnson Foundation asked communities and state health departments to develop a "childhood immunization monitoring and follow-up system," there was no commonly accepted definition of what was intended. The terms *monitoring system* (or *monitoring and follow-up system*), *tracking system,* and *registry system* have been used interchangeably by those developing the systems. The term *registry system* was once applied exclusively to the core database containing descriptive and demographic information on each child (usually derived from hospital birth records) and to which all immunization history was added when a child received immunizations. There is now a consensus that these systems can all be conveniently referred to as *registry systems* and defined this way:

> Manual or computer-based information systems by which to follow the immunization services provided to individual children in defined populations and to enable health care providers to ascertain (by computer or other means) the immunization status of individual children in a timely and accurate manner when immunization opportunities occur. Such systems should allow health care providers to input information on vaccines given at the point of service.[11]

Even before defining the terms "childhood immunization monitoring and follow-up systems," the Foundation requested proposals, appointed a national advisory committee to review them, conducted site visits, and selected an initial group of projects to receive planning grants.

In essence, the systems are intended to perform three basic functions. First, they identify children who are due or overdue for immunizations and notify parents, prompting them to make appointments for their children. Similarly, providers or outreach workers can be notified of missed immunizations for follow-up. Second, the systems provide a database for health care providers to monitor the immunization status of their patients as a reference point during patient encounters. By allowing all providers of child health services to enter immunization-related data into these systems, providers serving a particular child have a comprehensive information source available at the time they see a patient, no matter where a child may have received immunizations in the past. Third, these systems can provide a database to enable immunization program planners to identify populations at risk for delayed immunizations, to target interventions appropriately, and to evaluate the success of immunization efforts.

Defining the purpose and functions of an immunization registry system was an important step in the national effort to promote the development of these systems. Equally important is the effort to specify the key functional components of such systems. The national evaluation team, with assistance from the National Program Office and the CDC's National Immunization Program, sought to define the major functional expectations of such systems, realizing that many of the systems would address the issues in ways that would vary from approaches taken in other projects. The key functional components described in Exhibit 9.1 address capabilities expected of registry systems in four areas of activity: database, inputs, outputs, and system factors.

Most of the first generation of grantees reported the twenty-item list of key components to be useful in describing their registry systems. These criteria were never intended as a rigid set of expectations; rather, projects were expected to vary a great deal in the order in which they would address these functional task areas. However, there were expectations that at least some effort would be made in each of these twenty areas.

Registry System Sponsorship and Infrastructure

In most cases, local or state public health departments were the applicants for planning or implementation grants. It appears that they are often of pivotal importance and have the legal authority to address this important set of public health issues. The applicants hoped to involve private-sector providers of child health services—including individual physicians and group practices in pediatrics and family practice, community health centers, hospital clinics, and emergency rooms—in the registry systems. Although many public health departments have had interactions and cooperative arrangements with these entities in the past, the collaboration required to implement childhood

Exhibit 9.1.   Model Immunization Registry System Components.

Database

1. Includes all children in the selected age group.
2. Maintains records on children up through entry into school.
3. Includes the ability to monitor all immunizations recommended for children up to age two and can be modified to incorporate changes in recommendations.
4. Includes information needed to comply with school, state, and federal immunization reporting requirements. Such information might include vaccine type, date administered, site of injection, adverse reactions, and vaccine manufacturer and lot number.
5. Contains or can be linked to communicable disease information to identify and describe factors related to cases of vaccine-preventable diseases.

Inputs

6. Identifies neonates or infants at birth.
7. Contains related demographic data.
8. System allows input of immunization data from all providers either by direct entry or timely submission of entry-ready forms to a centralized data entry location.

Outputs

9. Provides access for all designated medical providers, allowing every provider to
   - Upload information on immunizations
   - Easily access a child's record to verify immunization status
10. Includes ability to notify parents before each immunization is due.
11. Includes ability to promptly notify parents, physicians, and/or outreach staff of missed immunizations.
12. Includes a plan for data analysis that is able to assess locality-specific, provider-specific, population-specific, and program-specific immunization status of children included in the monitoring system and provide feedback to these localities and providers with respect to the extent of coverage among populations served.
13. Includes provision for data outputs to support outreach activities to under-immunized groups of children.
14. Includes ability to identify alternative immunization providers, inform parents, and create a notice of referral for the parent's use in seeking services.

System factors

15. Has potential to expand to include additional health promotion/disease and injury prevention data such as lead screening and tuberculosis skin testing.
16. Provides for protection of confidential medical information by providing unique numeric identifiers, limiting access to the database, limiting data available for review, and complying with state laws and agency policies regarding sharing of medical information.
17. Includes appropriate incentives for participating in the system by providers and consumers.
18. Includes plan for financial support of the system over time.
19. System design is compatible with state and national monitoring and follow-up systems.
20. Includes a plan to evaluate the effectiveness and efficiency of the tracking system.

immunization registries may require a significantly higher degree of collaboration than ever before.

Although the emerging "community health information networks" (CHINs) tend to focus on inpatient care, these organizations may be able to take the lead in some communities as the emphasis of these systems shifts to include more ambulatory and managed care data. Some of them may be able to use their information-systems capability to handle the data-management aspects of local immunization registry systems. If they do, public health agencies or private-sector managed care organizations could perform the outreach needed to establish the registries.

At the time the All Kids Count initiative was beginning, there was a feeling that state and local immunization registries would lead to the creation of a *national* immunization registry system. This idea has since been discarded. It is unlikely that all communities will develop childhood immunization registry systems. Moreover, the challenges and costs associated with sustaining an enormous, constantly updated, and instantly interactive nationwide system are immense. This realization has led instead to a focus on the state and local levels as the appropriate places to house registries.

There are, however, important reasons to explore ways to link local or state registries for the purpose of creating national indicators of immunization coverage. The Subcommittee on Vaccination Registries of the National Vaccine Advisory Committee (NVAC), which reports to the U.S. Department of Health and Human Services, recommended the establishment of a "system of state-based registries that can be linked nationwide" in its 1994 report.[12] The sum of the information would yield state, and then national, estimates of immunization coverage. Local registry systems would be the principal source of immunization status data for child care providers.

Communities vary considerably, however, in the technical and financial resources available to implement and maintain an immunization registry system, and there is insufficient information by which to calculate the costs of such systems. Even in those projects assisted by The Robert Wood Johnson Foundation and other private philanthropies, it may not be easy to separate the costs of mounting an immunization registry project from the costs of maintaining other local public health immunization, information, and surveillance activities. It remains to be seen whether those public health agencies with substantial experience in epidemiological and other aspects of disease surveillance, or those with outreach programs designed to identify those adults, children, and families with greatest need for health services, have an advantage in the effort to develop immunization registries. Surveillance units of these agencies usually have persons with computer and data management skills as well as the computer equipment to implement a basic immunization registry effort. When these agencies have established mechanisms for integrating hospital birth records with records of existing public health outreach programs, they may be well positioned to develop key components of registry systems.

So far, it appears that local public agency management of immunization registries brings the best results. That said, there remains the problem of ensuring that these agencies have the necessary infrastructure to reach beyond their traditional boundaries and assume a role as coordinator of communitywide efforts in behalf of all children, regardless of their primary source of health care. Not only do these agencies need their own solid resource base; they must be able to draw upon the resources of private-sector health care organizations in these efforts.

Legislative Mandates to
Support Registry System Efforts

In a number of states and communities, including eight All Kids Count regions (Baltimore, New York City, California, Georgia, Philadelphia, Virginia, Mississippi, and Arizona), officials have acted under their public health authority to authorize or mandate immunization registries and/or the reporting of immunization events to a registry or to the public health authority.[13] In those communities, All Kids Count project directors have indicated that these regulations could facilitate their work. In other cities, registries are being developed without specific statutory authorization. While there is no current federal legislation requiring that these systems be developed, there are federal policies that support registry development; however, there is no single source of funding sufficient to develop them in every state and community. The collaboration of the public and private sectors at the national, state, and local levels continues to be essential. The fostering of public policy support of immunization registry and follow-up efforts may prove very helpful to their success but cannot substitute for energy and commitment at the community level.

Public- and Private-Sector Collaboration

One of the most difficult aspects of community-level efforts in developing childhood immunization registry systems concerns the participation of private-sector providers. Childhood immunization services vary widely from community to community. In many counties and cities of the American South and in California, the local health department is likely to serve as a major provider of direct primary care services to otherwise underserved and uninsured populations, but, with the exceptions of New York and New Jersey, this level of care would not be common among public health departments in the Northeast or the Midwest. In those regions, therefore, public health agencies may have very different ideas about how to achieve a central role in creating a community-based immunization registry system that involves both public- and private-sector providers. If both public- and private-sector providers do take part in developing an immunization registry, all children who use the health care system can be monitored and receive their immunizations on time. In some areas, a significant portion of the population may have limited contact with health care providers, public or private. In Mississippi, for example, the All Kids Count project staff members speculate that the 10 percent of children who are most difficult to reach, and those most likely to be underimmunized, simply do not seek health care of any kind. Immunization registries that use data from birth certificates as a base may be the most effective means of identifying this vulnerable population and ensuring that they receive not only vaccines but other primary care as well. (However, some All Kids Count registries are finding that birth certificate data can be inaccurate or incomplete and do not provide addresses through which parents can be reached.)

It is with regard to these children that immunization registries may have their greatest "value-added" impact. A child monitored through one of these registry systems can then be brought into contact with more general health care services. A child who comes in for a vaccination may well have other health needs that the health care provider can see to. If registry systems can be combined with an effective outreach program, access to primary health care in general can be improved.

There may be increased potential for this benefit with the widespread movement in the 1990s toward the delivery of services to Medicaid-eligible children through managed care contracts. Managed care organizations use immunization coverage rates as one indicator of the quality of services delivered under their plans, and this emphasis may bring about improved overall primary care for underimmunized children enrolled in both the immunization registry and the managed care plans.

During the early years of All Kids Count, managed care, including Medicaid managed care, increased in many areas of the nation. This environmental change has affected private practitioners and has brought about changes in the development of a number of the immunization registries. Grantees have begun to work out cooperative arrangements with managed care organizations so as to secure access to immunization updates and to bring their providers into the registries.

For their part, health plans across the country are demonstrating a corresponding interest in immunization registries. The 1996 Childhood Immunization Practices Survey, conducted by the American Association of Health Plans,[14] showed that more than 70 percent of those responding supported the concept of registry development, with particular interest in the ability to have access to data or to interface with the registries. The survey also indicated that 42 percent of 116 respondents were involved in some way in the development of registries by other organizations. More than half of the responding health plans reported having difficulty collecting immunization data from providers, and even more (69 percent) had difficulty acquiring data on immunizations given to children outside of their plans. Issues of concern cited by the health plans included the cost of registry development and participation, the potential for the unauthorized use of data, and the burden of data-entry requirements. Representatives of managed care organizations have voiced concerns that registry data (such as parents' names and addresses) might be used improperly to recruit clients from one health plan to another.

Technology Choice and Implementation

One of the most interesting elements in developing immunization registries involves the choice of a technological strategy. This choice is constrained by the availability of technical personnel, the interest and awareness among registry system and public health agency personnel of developments in information technology, the state of the art in medical and public health informatics, and the available financial resources to experiment with and adopt these technologies.

It is important to realize the complexity and level of administrative commitment that a comprehensive childhood immunization registry and follow-up system entails. In addition to maintaining a database updated from multiple sources, the systems must use the database to ensure that individual children are immunized. Systems must be in place that identify the immunization schedule for a child based on date of birth. Then these systems must be capable of providing prompts (to parents and providers) or must enable individual providers to do so for their patients. The number of events (clinical immunization encounters) such systems would have to track is usually five: (1) soon after birth; (2) at age two months; (3) age four months; (4) age six months; and (5) between fifteen and eighteen months.

For registry systems to send reminders both that immunizations are due *and* that immunizations are overdue (which is the case for more than half of the All Kids Count projects), this means a minimum of five notifications (to parents who have their children immunized on schedule) and a possible total of ten separate communications.

For children who receive their scheduled immunizations late or miss them, interventions must be designed, and these must involve collaboration with providers. Providers having experience with registries have found the "reminder" function of the registries to be worthwhile, as it can increase the percentage of scheduled—and kept—appointments and can stimulate parents to bring children for needed well-child care, not just for illnesses.

For an ongoing registry system to be cost-effective, the agencies operating the system must be prepared to analyze their databases over time in order to target populations or areas where underimmunization is most prevalent, and then design outreach efforts to provide services or interventions. Further, the advances in information technology that have made computer-based registry systems possible are continuing, and there are periodic costs associated with technology upgrades that have to take place from time to time. This has already been the case for one of the All Kids Count projects, which began with a commitment to a mainframe-based system and then had to make changes in technology and design in midcourse in order to interact with private providers. Obviously, this entailed substantial costs and staff time, in addition to delaying implementation of the registry.

Many All Kids Count registry projects have developed contractual relationships with private companies, such as software or systems design firms or in one case a university department, to obtain technical assistance needed in designing, staffing, and maintaining their systems. There can be an advantage, especially in the early stages, to having access to a substantial resource of additional expertise. However, there can be a loss of control; modifications can be more time-consuming when taken out-of-house, and if the contractual arrangement is not fulfilled by the outside contract organization, the project can be compromised. During the first three years of the All Kids Count program, several projects experienced delays related to difficulties with such outside organizations; in one case the resulting setbacks brought the project to a temporary, but very serious, halt. It seems certain that any collaborative or contractual arrangement is stronger where the agency responsible for the registry maintains both a high degree of commitment to the registry system effort and strong managerial control.

As the All Kids Count projects began to take shape, there was considerable interest in the application of new and often untested ideas for how computer-based technologies might augment the basic registry system efforts. Consideration was given to such technologies as "smart cards" (identification cards that can be read by machines for data entry and reimbursement information), patient-carried immunization records, computer-assisted telephone prompting, and online and fax-based systems for provider data input and querying.

The projects have recognized that a range of computer systems, both high-tech and low-tech, are necessary to permit users of the registries to supply and provide information. Most sites chose to build databases on powerful personal computers. A small number of projects, primarily among those based in larger areas, chose at least initially to build their databases on a mainframe computer. The form of database management and provider access most commonly selected was the client-server or file-server format, which permits users to conduct most of their interactions with the database on their own computers after having obtained the required files from the central server and which then allows them to return the updated or reviewed data to the central server for processing and storing. In this way some of the responsibility for database management is "distributed" among those generating the data.

The predominant early vision of these systems was based on the expectation that most providers would interact online with the registry using their office-based computers. That model has posed technological challenges, because providers have varying computer systems—or none at all—in their offices, and varying levels of in-house expertise and staff time. Accordingly, most projects have developed systems to accept and process periodic batch entries of computer data, submitted daily or perhaps weekly. Also, all of the projects have put in place systems to accept by mail or fax information sent to the registry and then entered centrally, or submitted over the telephone. Most have technologies allowing immunization information to be submitted over telephone lines to and from providers. This has involved establishing telephone lines, in some cases with toll-free numbers, and training registry staff to deal with telephone inquiries.

Projects have encountered problems getting consistently accurate and complete data from multiple providers, regardless of which technology is employed. Acquiring and maintaining a complete and accurate database has been a greater challenge than anticipated, even within an organized health department system. This problem can be compounded exponentially in settings where numerous private-sector physicians' offices or clinics provide immunization data updates, because these sites have varying in-house reporting systems, different computer systems, and differing degrees of staff commitment. Each provider organization participating in the registry must receive some form of training, either through instructional materials or on-site; staff turnover may result in untrained personnel submitting data, with the obvious potential for inaccuracies.

Security and Confidentiality

Support for the registries from providers, managed care organizations, and the general public rests in part on the ability to ensure the security and confidentiality of registry information. The All Kids Count project staffs have invested considerable effort in developing policies and procedures to protect individual privacy and prevent unauthorized or improper use of their records. These include methods to prevent "browsing" (viewing numerous records at one time), identify authorized users, and establish different levels of access based on the need to know.

At the outset of the All Kids Count initiative, there was much enthusiasm for the development of linkages between immunization data and other child health datasets. The original concept was to tie registry data to other relevant health data on a child so that more comprehensive primary care could be provided to children. For example, a provider seeing a child for the first time could, through linked or integrated datasets, learn that a child not only needed immunizations but was being followed for lead exposure. The provider could then determine if any further assessment was required. However, there have been many concerns about the advisability of such integrated databases, primarily for reasons of security and confidentiality. There are concerns that the nonimmunization data could be obtained and used improperly, for example by insurance companies that might choose to deny coverage.

About half of the All Kids Count projects have established or planned linkages to other data; those projects that are not linked tend to cite confidentiality as their primary reason for establishing stand-alone databases.

In most cases where databases have been or will be linked or integrated, they are linked only through the public health agency and primarily relate to public health programs such as WIC (a federally funded nutrition program for women, infants, and children) and lead screening. Only one registry system, still under development, envisions a more comprehensive child health database.

The issues of security and confidentiality, particularly of linked databases, remain very much on the agenda and continue to be of considerable importance as the data accumulate, the number of records increases, and more providers participate.

Area Size and Scope of Services

As the focus on local immunization registries has become clearer, the question of whether some communities are able to implement these systems arises; and, of course, some communities may have advantages associated with how delivery of local health services has developed. For example, in those communities with large numbers of Medicaid-eligible children and families, the advent of Medicaid managed care may make it easier to recruit private sector providers who participate in the registry through their affiliation with the health plans under contract to provide Medicaid services.

Community size and population density may affect the practicality of implementing computer-based information systems. In some rural counties where no more than half a dozen children in any birth cohort are scheduled for a particular immunization in a given month, there are concerns about the benefit to be gained from an investment in computer-generated reminders and overdue notices. A statewide registry might be particularly important in those states with many sparsely populated areas where the local population and public health infrastructure would not support multiple local registries. It may be that the outreach and follow-up efforts stimulated by the centralized registry database should vary by region; for example, outreach workers in less-populated areas might personally encourage parents to obtain immunizations for their children.

PROBLEMS AND PROSPECTS FOR THE FUTURE

The All Kids Count initiative can play a vital role in ensuring coverage levels of 90 percent or greater for two-year-old children by the year 2000 *and sustaining* those levels thereafter. History has shown that once a crisis is over, memories of low immunization levels and disease outbreaks subside, and immunization rates may drop again, only to be followed by further outbreaks and their human and societal costs. The All Kids Count registries represent an important approach to maintaining high immunization levels regardless of the ebb and flow of public awareness. By institutionalizing these programs (including both monitoring of immunization status and outreach efforts), there is greater likelihood that recent gains can be sustained.

All of the All Kids Count registries funded by The Robert Wood Johnson Foundation are expected to be operational by the end of 1997, although several that have experienced delays may not be as fully implemented as originally anticipated. By the year 2000, most will have monitored the immunization levels of at least two annual cohorts of two-year-old children who were registered in these information systems at the time of birth. These systems will have the ability to sustain high levels of immunization in the communities they serve, and to document their results.

One lesson has emerged from these efforts so far: few very important public health accomplishments occur without broad-based, multisectoral collaboration and strategic investment of sufficient resources. A substantial investment by government, nongovernmental organizations, and corporations has brought about the highest recorded level of early childhood immunizations to date—concrete evidence that the nation's health can be protected through the use of the vaccines and the childhood vaccination schedules that medical science has so painstakingly developed. We have not yet reached our goals; although there are a number of registries in operation or under development, thanks in great part to the All Kids Count initiative, many more communities are at best in the planning stages of registry development or not yet considering it. Although the states are continuing to develop plans, there is considerable variation in their rates of progress.

As the CDC continues to work with states to develop plans for local or statewide registries, the experiences of the All Kids Count projects appear to have been beneficial. In the fall of 1996, the CDC produced first drafts of extensive guidelines for immunization registry and follow-up systems. The guidelines were produced by a group that included a number of representatives of the All Kids Count projects and the national program office in Atlanta; the documents bear the names of the CDC and All Kids Count as cosponsors. The National Vaccine Advisory Committee promptly endorsed the section addressing confidentiality, which related to the issues that were of most immediate concern to it.

Additionally, through annual national and regional meetings, the All Kids Count projects promoted and supported the development of immunization registries. The meetings were open to and well attended by participants from many other locations. Thus, the linkages among registries that are not yet technically feasible may have begun informally and unofficially. It remains to be seen whether the function served by these meetings can be carried forward under other sponsorship when foundation funding ends.

In any event, the All Kids Count initiative has played a role in setting national policy for the development of immunization registry and follow-up systems. The experiences of the All Kids Count projects have shown that the task is a complex one, requiring technical expertise, careful administrative oversight, and long-term participation by the providers of childhood immunizations.

Endnotes

1. National Vaccine Advisory Committee, "The Measles Epidemic: The Problems, Barriers, and Recommendations," *JAMA* 266 (1991), 1547–1552; W. L. Atkinson, W. A. Orenstein, and S. Krugman, "The Resurgence of

Measles in the United States, 1989–1994," *Annual Review of Medicine,* 43 (1992), 451–463.

2. Centers for Disease Control and Prevention, "The National Immunization Program (NIP) Overview. Immunization for All Ages/Immunization: A Lifetime Commitment," 30th Annual Immunization Conference, Washington, D.C., Apr. 9–12, 1996, pp. 1–5.

3. Centers for Disease Control and Prevention, "National, State, and Urban Area Vaccination Coverage Levels Among Children Aged 19–35 Months: United States, April 1994–March 1995," *Morbidity and Mortality Weekly Report* 45(7) (Feb. 23, 1996), 145–150.

4. Centers for Disease Control and Prevention, "Vaccination Coverage of 2–year-old Children: United States, January–March 1994," *MMWR* 44 (1995), 142–143, 149–150. Summarized in L. O. Gostin and Z. Lazzarini, "Childhood Immunization Registries: A National Review of Public Health Information Systems and the Protection of Privacy," *JAMA* 274 (1995), 1793–1799.

5. D. Satcher, "Keep up the Progress on Childhood Immunization," *Public Health Reports* 109(5) (1994), 593.

6. D. L. Wood, R. A. Hayward, C. R. Corey, H. E. Freeman, and M. F. Shapiro, "Access to Medical Care for Children and Adolescents in the United States," *Pediatrics* 86 (1990), 666–673.

7. A. Skolnick, "Should Insurance Cover Routine Immunizations?" *JAMA* 265 (1991), 2453–2457.

8. L. E. Rodewald, "Public Health in Private Practice: The Challenge of Immunizing Preschool Children," *Public Health Management and Practice* 2 (1996), vii–viii.

9. U.S. General Accounting Office, *CDC's National Immunization Survey; Methodological Problems Limit Survey's Utility: Report to the Honorable Dale Bumpers, U.S. Senate* (Sept. 1996), P. 20.

10. Robert Wood Johnson Foundation, *All Kids Count: Establishing Immunization Monitoring and Follow-up Systems (Call for Proposals)* (Princeton, N.J.: author, 1991), p. 3.

11. Robert Wood Johnson Foundation, All Kids Count. *Childhood Immunization Registry Systems: A General Definition of Terms, Scope, and Components* (Princeton, N.J.: author, 1996) p. 5.

12. National Vaccine Advisory Committee, *Developing a National Childhood Immunization Information System: Registries, Reminders, and Recall* (Washington, D.C.: Subcommittee on Vaccination Registries, U.S. Department of Health and Human Services, U.S. Public Health Service, 1994).

13. L. O. Gostin and Z. Lazzarini, "Childhood Immunization Registries: A National Review of Public Health Information Systems and the Protection of Privacy," *JAMA* 274 (1995), 1793–1799.

14. Medical Affairs Department, American Association of Health Plans, "Report from the 1996 Survey of Health Plan Immunization Practices," *Childhood Immunization Newsletter* (July/Aug. 1996), 4–5.

CHAPTER TEN

—⁓— The Homeless Families Program

A Summary of Key Findings

Debra J. Rog
Marjorie Gutman

Editors' Introduction

The Foundation has made two investments in large national programs directed at alleviating problems facing homeless people in America. The first, Health Care for the Homeless, attempted to increase the availability of health care services for homeless people. It became a model that was cited when the federal government passed the McKinney Act in 1987, providing federal dollars to improve access to health care for homeless people throughout the country.

After the Health Care for the Homeless program was completed, the Foundation funded a second program, this time focusing on homeless *families*. The Homeless Families Program was more ambitious than the first. It attempted to improve not only health care services for homeless families but also a range of other social services generally important to their well-being. The Foundation entered an active and productive partnership with the federal Department of Housing and Urban Development, which made stable housing arrangements available to the families participating in the program.

The premise of the program was that both housing and social services (including health care) were needed to get many homeless families back into stable and independent life circumstances.

The Homeless Families Program exemplifies a range of national programs begun by the Foundation in the late 1980s and the start of the 1990s, which emphasized systems reform as a long-range solution to making public investments in social services more productive. The theory held that the problem with social services was not just that more were necessary but that existing resources needed to be better coordinated and better focused.

Chapter Ten was written by Debra J. Rog and Marjorie Gutman. They present findings from the formal evaluation of the program that the Foundation funded soon after the program was initiated. This chapter offers insights into the problems faced by homeless families as well as the obstacles faced by program managers trying to bring about system reform. The discussion also addresses the challenges involved in designing and implementing "enriched services" accompanying housing for the homeless.

Rog, who is a research fellow at the Center for Mental Health Policy, Institute for Public Policy Studies at Vanderbilt University, has published extensively on the problems of homelessness in America. Gutman, a senior program officer of the Foundation who was in charge of the design and monitoring of this evaluation, has been active in developing and evaluating a number of Foundation programs addressing the needs of vulnerable populations.

Americans have a short attention span. A newly discovered problem receives major national attention from the public and policy makers for a few years, only to be replaced by another pressing problem. Most disturbing, in the case of social issues, the first problem is rarely resolved and the "new" one may even be another manifestation of the same issue.

This is certainly true of homelessness. During the 1980s, homelessness took center stage as a largely unexpected new problem for our society. Homeless people have been found in most times and places, of course, but the increasing appearance of homeless women and children, and even whole families, on the streets and in shelters made the issue highly visible and compelling.[1] Best estimates were that women and children totaled one-fifth to one-third of the homeless population.[2] One heated debate at the time concerned the extent to which these families were homeless because of temporary economic dislocation or because of endemic poverty and other complicating factors.

It was against this backdrop that the *Homeless Families Program,* a five-year effort, was initiated in 1990. Even as the HFP was starting, national attention on homelessness was already beginning to wane and has remained low ever since. It is true that a small cadre of activists, providers, policy makers, and dedicated volunteers have continued to grapple with the problem, and it does surface now and again in public debate. But by and large the public's attention is captured by current concerns—welfare reform, the "underclass," violence—and it is easy to forget that homeless persons, and especially homeless families, are a small but very important part of the "new" problems the nation is trying to address.

PROGRAM OVERVIEW

The Homeless Families Program, a joint effort of The Robert Wood Johnson Foundation and the Department of Housing and Urban Development, was the first large-scale response to the problem of family homelessness. Started in nine cities across the nation, it had two complementary goals:

1. To develop or restructure the systems of health, support services, and housing for families

2. To develop a model of *services-enriched housing* for families who have multiple, complex problems

The ultimate goal of the Homeless Families Program was to improve the residential stability of families, promote greater use of services, and increase steps toward self-sufficiency. In addition, as a demonstration program the HFP integrated a major evaluation into the initiative at all sites. The evaluation was designed to learn more about the needs of families who struggle with homelessness and other problems, to learn how services and systems might be better organized and delivered to meet those needs, and to examine how housing might be delivered to promote stability and use of services as well as progress toward self-sufficiency.

The Homeless Families Program was an outgrowth of several previous demonstration programs. One main progenitor was the nineteen–city Health Care for the Homeless Program, cofunded by The Robert Wood Johnson Foundation and the Pew Charitable Trusts in 1985.[3] Under this program, thousands of homeless people received health services, assessments, and referrals through primary care clinics located in shelters. The simple premise of the program was to make health care accessible to homeless people by locating it where they congregate and by tailoring the care to their special needs. The program accomplished its goal of demonstrating the feasibility and the acceptability of health clinics for homeless persons, and it became the template for the hundreds of clinics supported in many cities under the 1987 Stewart B. McKinney Act—the nation's landmark legislation in homelessness.

Additionally, evaluation of the Health Care for the Homeless Program led to the first large multicity dataset on the characteristics of homeless people and their health care needs. This study, along with others conducted at the time, helped establish the fact that young families—consisting mostly of single women with two to three children—made up a significant segment, and the fastest-growing one, of the homeless population.[4] These studies also documented that members of homeless families were experiencing significant health problems, depression, and developmental delays. For example, roughly 33 percent of homeless mothers in the study suffered from psychiatric problems, and roughly 20 percent abused alcohol or illegal drugs. The children in these situations had very low rates of immunization and suffered from extraordinarily high rates of childhood illness. Thirty-five percent of them had recurrent ear infections. The incidence of chronic disorders ran approximately twice the norm. Finally, data from the Health Care for the Homeless Program supported the contention of many researchers that a significant number of these children were at risk for long-term, if not permanent, developmental delay.

Growing recognition and evidence of the more complex needs of subgroups of the homeless, especially these families, led to the development of the Homeless Families Program. The design of the HFP reflects experiences from yet another Robert Wood Johnson Foundation/HUD joint initiative, the Program on Chronic Mental Illness, as well as HUD's Transitional Housing Program under the McKinney Act. Both of these programs reinforced the view that although permanent housing was absolutely necessary, it was not in itself sufficient if substantial segments of the homeless population were to achieve stability and self-sufficiency. Rather, these individuals and families appeared to need more comprehensive, individually tailored benefits involving permanent housing, health, social, and support services. The Program on Chronic Mental Illness,[5] an effort to create more centralized local systems of care, also furthered the view that, in addition to new ways of delivering services, systemic efforts were needed to help vulnerable populations.

Thus, the first premise of the Homeless Families Program is that whereas some families are homeless for reasons that are primarily economic, others face more complex problems. For them, a lack of housing was not believed to be the sole cause of their homelessness, and housing alone was not the simple solution to it. Such families might need continuing and comprehensive health, housing, and supportive services in order to function in the community. The second premise is that these families need case management to help them get necessary services. Public funding has made a number of services and supports available to young families, through Aid to Families with Dependent Children; Medicaid; Maternal and Child Health; the Supplemental Food Program for Women, Infants, and Children (WIC); Social Service Block Grants; Head Start; and the McKinney Act funds. But these services are fragmented among agencies and may be difficult for homeless mothers to obtain.

The third premise is that although a number of communities do provide many of the services available for homeless families, these efforts are splintered, and a more systemic approach is needed. A modest infusion of grant money and housing subsidies could enable these communities to build comprehensive, coordinated service systems to ensure that these young families get the continuing services they need.

Each of the nine HFP sites received approximately $600,000 in grant money over five years to facilitate systems of care for homeless families and, within that context, to demonstrate a model of services-enriched housing for a group of families. The projects were led by either a city or a county public agency, a coalition or task force for the homeless, or another nonprofit provider. Guided by the HFP National Program Office and HUD, each project developed a memorandum of understanding with the local public housing authority. Through this agreement, each project received an allotment of approximately 150 Section 8 housing certificates[6] from HUD to allocate to families with multiple problems, many of whom had not been on the existing waiting list of the public housing authority. For each family receiving a Section 8 certificate, the HFP lead agency was to provide or obtain services through case management. Robert Wood Johnson Foundation support of the program totaled $4.7 million, while HUD's contribution totaled $30 million in rental subsidies over five years.

EVALUATION DESCRIPTION

An evaluation was designed to answer three major questions:

1. What is the nature of the system initiatives and specific services-enriched housing interventions implemented in each of the projects?

2. What is the nature of the target population served in the Homeless Families Program?

3. What are the outcomes of the system initiatives and the specific services-enriched housing interventions for the service systems and for the families participating in the initiatives?[7]

Preliminary results of the evaluation are reported below.

DESCRIPTION OF PARTICIPATING FAMILIES

Of the 1,670 families accepted into the program and included in its management information system, 1,298 entered services-enriched housing. These families, the focus of the evaluation, were similar demographically to families described in other studies of homeless families and welfare recipients. The average family was headed by a woman in her late twenties or early thirties, with two children, at least one of whom was less than three years old. Ethnicity and education varied across the sites, most often reflecting the characteristics of the particular site. Service needs appeared to be more pervasive and severe for the HFP families than has been the case in other studies of homeless families and families receiving welfare.[8]

EVALUATION FINDINGS

Families: Needs, Strengths, and Outcomes

Because the program targeted homeless families with multiple problems, there are limitations to the extent to which these data can be applied to the full population of homeless families. However, the results do clarify the complexity and the character of a segment of the population and help anchor an understanding of the broader population. Perhaps most important, taken together with the outcomes, we can learn what is possible even for families with the most complex challenges and needs.

FAMILIES IN NEED OFTEN PRESENT A WEB OF INTERRELATED AND DEEP-SEATED CHALLENGES.   Families served through the HFP struggled with homelessness and residential instability for some time. On average, families experienced their first time without their own home about five years before they entered the program. In the eighteen months just before entering the HFP, most of the families spent time either in a shelter (approximately five months) or doubled up (five months). Families spent about seven months in their own homes, but rarely consecutively. The families moved frequently—about every three and half months in the eighteen-month period—before entering the HFP.

Housing instability is only one of the areas of difficulty for the families who entered the program. All areas of need were pronounced (Table 10.1) for the population of women served, especially in comparison to the general population. Additionally, the majority of families had multiple service needs in the areas of physical and mental health, substance abuse, education and training, and others. In fact, nearly a quarter were found to have current needs in all three major areas examined—human capital, physical health, and mental health-related—and 80 percent had needs in two or more categories.

Table 10.1   Indicators of Strengths and Needs of HFP Mothers* (767 Families).

Human Capital	% of HFP Mothers
Having high school/GED or greater at intake	58
Held the same job for one year or more before intake	62

Health	
Reporting two or more health problems in past year	26
Having a health rating of fair or poor	31

Mental Health-Related	
Mental Health	
Psychologically distressed	59
Ever hospitalized for mental health	15
Hospitalized for mental health in past year	3
Ever attempted suicide	28
Attempted suicide in past year	2
Any childhood risk factor**	58
Alcohol and Drugs	
"Alcoholic"	29
Ever used hard drugs	49
Used hard drugs in past year	12
Domestic Violence	
Current partner violence	18
Past partner violence	81

* Data are from the Family Assessment, an in-depth interview conducted with families housed at least four months. Approximately 65 percent of the eligible families across the sites completed assessments, and of these, approximately 95 percent were completed by women and included in this analysis. The number of women completing each question varies. Standardized measures on the assessment include excerpts from the National Health and Nutrition Examination Survey (HANES) and a modified version of the Health Interview Schedule (HIS), the Center for Epidemiologic Studies Depression Scale (CES-D), the Short Michigan Alcoholism Screening Test (SMAST), and a modified Conflict Tactics Scale (CTS) measure of domestic violence. See D. J. Rog, K. L. McCombs-Thornton, A. M. Gilbert-Mongelli, C. Brito, and C. S. Holupka, "Implementation of the Homeless Families Programs: Characteristics, Strengths, and Needs of Participant Families," *American Journal of Orthopsychiatry* 65(4) (1995), 514–528, for a more detailed description of the Family Assessment.

** Childhood risk factors include placement in foster care, running away for a week or longer, and experiencing severe physical abuse or sexual abuse as a child.

MENTAL HEALTH NEEDS AND DOMESTIC VIOLENCE SURFACE AS TWO DIS-ABLING FACTORS FOR THE FAMILIES. Perhaps the most marked areas of need that these women have tackled through much of their lives fall within the category of mental health. Even as children, more than half of them would have been considered at risk for future mental health problems because they had been placed in foster care, had run away for a week or longer, or had experienced physical and/or sexual abuse.

As adults, the vast majority of women in the HFP had one or more indications of mental health need. A sizable percentage, 15 percent, were hospitalized one or more times for a mental health problem, 3 percent in the year before they came into the program. More than half were considered psychologically distressed and in need of further evaluation for depression.

One of the most troubling findings in this area is the extent to which these women have been victims of abuse and, in turn, have tried to hurt themselves. Nearly all (81 percent) reported some type of abuse by a former partner, and 65 percent reported one or more severe acts of violence by a past partner. In addition, more than a third cited domestic violence as a reason for moving in the five years before they entered the program.

Reports of suicide attempts by these women were almost ten times as frequent as they were for the general population (28 percent versus 3 percent). Of those who reported ever attempting suicide, more than half of this group—57 percent—reported multiple attempts. Drug overdosing was the most common method used. The seriousness of the suicide attempts is highlighted by the fact that 43 percent of the most recent attempts resulted in a hospitalization and, in fact, account for the majority of the mental health hospitalizations reported.

THROUGH THEIR PARTICIPATION IN THE HFP, FAMILIES INCREASE THEIR ACCESS TO AND USE OF AN ARRAY OF SERVICES. A critical discovery made as families entered the Homeless Families Program was that the majority of them were not receiving needed services.[9] In fact, the vast majority—70 percent or more of those in need—were not receiving mental health, dental, and alcohol treatment services. A smaller but still sizable percentage of families, 58 percent, were not receiving needed drug services.

Through the program, access to services appeared to improve (Table 10.2). The biggest increases were experienced in mental health services, followed by alcohol and drug services. Because families had reported relatively high access before they entered the HFP, health services did not change while they were in the program. Access to dental services increased slightly, but adult family members continued to have a high level of unmet need.[10]

FAMILIES ACROSS THE SITES HAVE MADE CONSIDERABLE GAINS IN RESIDENTIAL STABILITY. Despite years of instability, families achieved substantial residential stability after they entered the program. At eighteen months after entering the program, more than 85 percent of the families were still stably housed in the six sites that provided data. This represents more than a *doubling* of the time the families spent in permanent housing for the same period before they entered the program. The remainder of families either lost their Section 8 certificate because of one or more violations—fraud, for example—or voluntarily returned the certificate (for example, to move to another state).

After thirty months, rates of stability continued to be high, but more differences emerged among program sites. In three of the six sites for which data are available, more than 80 percent of the families were known to be in permanent housing, typically with the original Section 8 certificates. In the other three sites, fewer than 65 percent were known to be residentially stable in permanent housing. Analyses to date have identified few stable predictors of housing loss within and across sites. When the data are examined through the use of more complex statistical analysis, they show that the loss of housing is related to mothers' reports of current severe violence as well as being pregnant or having an infant at the time they entered the program.[11] These two predictors are important and troubling, and both will continue to be explored in future analyses.

Table 10.2   Service Needs and Access.

	% of HFP Families Needing Each Service	% Receiving:	
		At Intake	At Least Once While in Program
Health	83	76	73
Mental Health	68	29	64
Dental	62	30	38
Alcohol Services	50	28	58
Drug Services	51	42	61

FAMILIES HAVE MADE LITTLE AND ERRATIC PROGRESS TOWARD SELF-
SUFFICIENCY AND CONTINUE TO HAVE CONSIDERABLE DEPENDENCE ON
FEDERAL AND STATE SUPPORT. Participation in education, job training,
and employment has fluctuated throughout the Homeless Families
Program. The data from the management information system do not
permit a sensitive and complete analysis of the changes in these areas,
but for those sites where data are available, it appears that about 40 percent of the primary parents have attended school at least once during
the program, and about half received some employment or vocational
service, including counseling and job training. About half of the primary parents also reported working some time during this period.

When families leave the program, having received a year or so of
case management services, 20 percent of the primary parents are
known to be working, compared with 13 percent when they entered.[12]
The increase is slight and not uniform, which means that some individuals who were employed when they entered the program were not
working when they left it. Although some sites showed increases in
the number of people with jobs, in most cases the increases were not
statistically significant. In addition, a few reportedly had a job lined
up (5 percent); about 9 percent were in job training, and 16 percent
reported being in school. Taken together, 39 percent were working,
preparing to work, or obtaining further education.

A number of factors may explain the unstable movement toward
self-sufficiency shown by most families in the HFP. One factor is that
the projects focused more on helping families remain residentially stable than on becoming self-sufficient; another is that a year or so after
entry into the program may still be too early to determine accurately
how successful a family will be at self-sufficiency. Indeed, residential
stability and self-sufficiency may go hand in hand, since part of the
rationale behind the program is that residential stability is required
before anyone in a family can begin to think about holding a full-time
job, continuing schooling, and moving off public assistance. Even after
thirty months, the data on residential stability indicate that the vast
majority of families who remain in permanent housing were still receiving subsidies, and the available information on those who returned
the Section 8 certificates or lost them suggests that these families were
most likely in unstable living and working situations. Few appeared
to have moved off public assistance, and very few off Section 8.

Lack of child care may be a major barrier to achieving self-sufficiency.
Across the sites, 72 percent of the families in the program were

reported to need child care services at intake and/or during the program. Only 41 percent of the families needing child care services were reported to have received them at least once throughout the program.

It is also important to recognize the range and the magnitude of the problems faced by most of the families in the HFP. Their past lives often have been challenged by economic and personal traumas. Even though the data suggest that the HFP has given them access to some services, many of the problems are long-standing and unlikely to disappear instantly. Despite increased housing stability, many families remain vulnerable to the ordinary challenges of life, let alone to broader reforms. The primary parents in these families often cycle through jobs, education, and services in response to other events in their lives—reuniting with a former batterer, for instance, or returning to drug or alcohol abuse. The overwhelming majority of HFP families received multiple public benefits (AFDC, food stamps, school lunches) and were likely to be substantially affected by changes in welfare and related benefit programs. Whether the new programs can adequately prepare these families to enter the workforce within the time frame stipulated remains to be seen. Families' involvement in similar efforts in the past appear to have limited benefit, at least in the short run.

Systems

The evaluation was designed to examine how service systems can be developed, organized, and sustained to respond to the needs of homeless families, especially those with multiple needs.

THE SERVICE "SYSTEM" FOR HOMELESS FAMILIES IS ILL-DEFINED AND FRAGMENTED AND INVOLVES MULTIPLE SERVICES AND SYSTEMS.   In fact, the term *homeless system* is a misnomer; for families in particular, there are often multiple systems that provide services. Each of these systems has its own level of fragmentation, and the connections among the various systems are even looser.

Three types of service systems are relevant to homeless families: homeless services, mainstream services, and coordinating services. Homeless services are specifically designed for individuals and families who lack a regular and permanent place to stay. In most places, these services include shelter and transitional housing, as well as food, clothing, and furniture assistance.

Mainstream services refer to those needed by most low-income families, homeless or otherwise. These include housing, income support, child care, health and dental care, mental health services, counseling for domestic violence, alcohol and drug treatment, and others. Many mainstream service systems are well established but were not designed to serve a homeless population. An examination of the systems across the nine HFP sites revealed few absolute gaps in services for homeless families. Every site had some type of child care available, for example, and some form of mental health services. What was more common and amazingly consistent across the sites were gaps in specific types of services resulting from limitations in capacity, eligibility restrictions, high costs, and constraints on accessibility. This finding conflicted with a key program premise, that services for homeless families did exist.

Common service gaps include affordable housing, with a desperate need for larger units and subsidies to ensure affordability; residential alcohol and drug programs that permit mothers to keep their children with them; affordable child care; mental health services for adults and children who are not seriously and persistently mentally ill but are trying to cope with issues of domestic violence, depression, and other problems stemming from their past instability; general legal assistance; and dental services for adults beyond extractions and fillings. Often, transportation is not available or not affordable, which creates an additional barrier to services.

Coordination services for families, if available, typically entail some form of case management. When case management was available in shelters and transitional housing, it was generally in short supply and of limited duration, with little if any follow-up once a family moved into permanent housing. Some mainstream services, such as job training, had case management attached to them, but it was also generally of limited duration and involved only services brokering. At the HFP sites, case management was not routinely available to homeless families moving into permanent housing. Therefore, unless families were in the HFP, they were largely on their own to negotiate the web of systems and services when they moved into permanent housing.

THE HFP HAS LED TO SOME FIXING OF THE SYSTEM. A goal of the HFP was to change the systems for dealing with the homeless. By and large, however, the system activities of the HFP projects did not result in broad-based changes but rather in some temporary or small-scale fix to improve service delivery for the families needing the service. The most common HFP system activities were project fixes: filling service gaps for the families in the HFP services-enriched housing. Mental health services, for example, were a critical gap for families participating in the program. Unable to obtain timely access for families needing therapy and other services to cope with the effects of domestic violence or other problems, a number of the HFP sites responded by hiring individual therapists to work with their families. The HFP efforts thus improved the accessibility of mental health services for families in the project, but they did not change how the overall mental health system relates to homeless families.

Other HFP activities created "system fixes" in which services were increased or improved for homeless families other than those in the demonstration. For example, the HFP National Program Office developed ways to use the Federally Qualified Health Center provision of Medicaid to create additional resources to cover the costs of case management and other services. This typically involved working with a single community health center or a Health Care for the Homeless clinic. Although the effort had the potential to spread systemwide, it was relatively circumscribed and independent of other reforms within the health care system.

System changes—enduring and far-reaching reformulations or modifications in the structure of a system—were rare in the Homeless Families Program. The one exception involved changes in the role of the public housing authority. Through their participation in the program, several housing authorities increased their awareness of, and sensitivity to, the needs of homeless families. They became more active participants in developing supportive housing for this population. The efforts of The Robert Wood Johnson Foundation and HUD appear to have been key factors in facilitating this change.

THE COMPLEXITY AND THE FRAGMENTATION OF SERVICE SYSTEMS FOR FAMILIES TRANSITIONING FROM HOMELESSNESS MAKES TRUE CHANGE DIFFICULT, IF NOT IMPOSSIBLE, FOR SMALL PRIVATE INITIATIVES. Although ambitious, the efforts of the Homeless Families Program to reform systems were in many ways overpowered by the complexity of the systems that needed restructuring. First, restructuring systems to meet the needs of homeless families meant dealing not with just one system but with several systems. Most of these systems are large and complex and serve a variety of people, of whom homeless families generally make up a small and relatively invisible fraction. Significant changes in mainstream systems are unlikely to be driven by the needs of this subpopulation of clients.

Second, the positioning of the Homeless Families Program in each community rarely gave it the clout needed to restructure or build a homeless service system. In some cases, the HFP was a program within a city or county health agency. At best, it could call upon the agency leadership to coordinate the efforts of other agencies. In other cases, the program was located in coalitions or task forces for the homeless that might have had the influence to bring groups together and to *identify* needed changes but were not in a position to *make* the changes happen.

Third, the resources that the HFP brought to the communities were too small to allow for major restructuring. The modest funding provided to each site was used to support a program director and case management or program staff. Although the Section 8 certificates contributed from HUD for this initiative were not inconsequential, they were designated as housing subsidies, not flexible funds that could be used to create new systems or strategies for action. Ironically, just having these certificates caused projects to focus much of their limited resources on the development and implementation of the services-enriched housing and less on the more nebulous goal of creating systems change.

SYSTEMS CHANGE AT THE LOCAL LEVEL MAY BE SPURRED BY FEDERAL AND NATIONAL LEADERSHIP. The one area where systems change appeared most consistently involved the public housing authorities. Across the sites, the housing authorities became stronger and more vocal participants in supportive housing for families. In addition to providing concrete advice that spurred collaboration between housing authorities and the HFP lead agencies, HUD and the Foundation required them to work out a Memorandum of Understanding. The framework for these memoranda, developed by HUD and the HFP National Office, stipulated the nature of collaboration that was expected between the housing authority and the HFP over the five years of the program. The memorandum was often used, particularly in the early stages of the program, as a tool to prod the housing authorities to modify procedures, cut red tape, and institute other changes needed to get the program off the ground. In addition, by having a written memorandum, the projects were less susceptible to internal changes (such as changes in executive directors of the housing authorities) that could otherwise threaten the agency's involvement in the HFP.

THE ABILITY TO ENGINEER AND MEASURE SYSTEMS CHANGE IS HAMPERED BY THE LACK OF A THEORY OF SYSTEMS CHANGE.   The Homeless Families Program had no articulated theory of systems change. Absent from the projects was a perspective of what the ideal system should be for families in order to break the cycle of homelessness. The goals were nonspecific, and the steps needed to achieve the goals were not detailed. None of the projects was preceded by an assessment of the needs, gaps, and strengths in the system. To fill this gap, the evaluation developed a framework of the ideal system to use as a tool for benchmarking the varied activities of the sites.

In addition, there was no explicit strategy for bringing about change. The desired outcome was a system that would be coordinated, accessible, and comprehensive. The general thinking was that the projects would work with other agencies to determine the changes that were needed in the current system, and either reorganize it or identify and leverage additional resources for new and enhanced services, or both. Ironically, the one very positive initiative, the Memorandum of Understanding, was not consciously viewed as a vehicle for systems change but as a mechanism to ensure that the Section 8 certificates would be dedicated to this program. The system changes stimulated by the memoranda were an unexpected by-product.

Services

The evaluation was also designed to provide a detailed look at the implementation of services-enriched housing. Little is known about how best to meet the needs of families who have been homeless and have had other problems for years. One of the more widely touted strategies has been to provide services, particularly case management, to families for some period of time after they move to permanent housing. The Homeless Families Program was the first large-scale attempt to provide services-enriched permanent housing to families. HUD's Shelter+Care and Supportive Housing Programs, which also combine case management services and housing, are a major part of HUD's continuum-of-care strategy for homeless families and individuals. Despite the increasing use of case management, there has been little explicit study of its effectiveness with homeless families. The HFP provided an unparalleled opportunity to study case management and other key aspects of services-enriched housing.

DESPITE A COMMON MODEL OF INTERVENTION, THE AMOUNT OF CASE MANAGEMENT PROVIDED TO HOMELESS FAMILIES VARIES DRAMATI-CALLY.   There was a remarkable similarity in the background and training of the case managers hired at the nine HFP sites, in the types of activities they conducted, and in the services they provided.[13] The vast majority of case managers working in this program were women in their thirties or forties, with a bachelor's or higher degree in social work or a related field, who had been working as case managers for five or fewer years. Most reported that their time with families was spent arranging services, making routine visits or calls to families, and working with families on skills development issues, such as budgeting or problem solving.

Despite the similarities, the differences in the amount of case management provided to families are striking. Although the average family received fifteen hours of contact during their first twelve months in the program, 33 percent of the families received less than six hours, whereas nearly 20 percent received more than twenty-four hours, and 5 percent received more than fifty hours.[14]

Sites differed greatly with respect to the intensity of the case management offered; statistically they can be grouped into four levels. At the high end, families at one site received an average of fifty-two hours of case management during their first year in the program, or about an hour a week. All the other sites had relatively less intensive case management, with case managers in most projects meeting with each family about one hour every two to three weeks. In two sites, families met with their case manager less than one hour a month.

IMPLEMENTING INTENSIVE CASE MANAGEMENT FOR HOMELESS FAMILIES REQUIRES A DIFFERENT APPROACH THAN THAT USED IN THE HFP.   Intensive case management was to be one of the cornerstones of the Homeless Families Program, with case managers spending as much time as needed with families. Although no explicit definition of intensive case management was provided, it was generally understood to mean at least one hour a week of face-to-face contact with each family. A key insight gained from this evaluation is that even when the HFP projects were implemented as designed—a caseload of one manager to twenty families, working with families a year or longer, visiting families in their home—the expected level of intensity could not be achieved.

With the need to spend time on paperwork, phone calls, meetings, travel, and so on, case managers spent little over an hour *a month* with each family, and they generally had one-quarter of the day to meet face-to-face with families. Assuming a one-to-twenty caseload, only if case managers had at least half of each day to meet with families could they reach the program goal of an hour a week in direct contact with each family. In order to achieve the desired level of intensity, the caseload and the work responsibility of case workers needs to be reduced, and they should be teamed with lay helpers and other support mechanisms.

INDIVIDUALS SKILLED IN LOCATING HOUSING AND WORKING WITH LAND-LORDS MAY BE AN IMPORTANT SERVICE FOR FAMILIES WHO HAVE NOT HAD PREVIOUS SUCCESS WITH HOUSING, ESPECIALLY IN TIGHT HOUSING MAR-KETS.   An innovation at several project sites was the appointment of a housing locator. This person identifies promising housing, recruits landlords, helps families find housing, and performs other related activities. A locator has typically been used at sites where the low-income housing market is especially tight and landlords willing to take Section 8 certificates are not numerous. For most of the public housing authorities, this position was new and welcome; in at least one site, the housing locator was continued within the housing authority so that he could work directly with any family needing assistance. At another site where the housing market was beginning to tighten over the last year of the HFP, the housing authority was seriously exploring the possibilities of hiring a housing locator to help families find landlords willing to take HUD Section 8 certificates.

IMPLICATIONS OF THE EVALUATION FINDINGS FOR HOMELESS FAMILIES AND BEYOND

The findings outlined below are pertinent not only for initiatives directed toward homeless families but also for a broader set of initiatives aimed at building and changing systems.

1.   *Systems building requires a theory of systems change and an understanding of the systems that exist and that are desired.* The HFP

system efforts might have been more successful if a study of the nature of the service systems involved had been conducted before the program started and a detailed theory of how to affect change had been developed. The program was initiated at sites where project directors had little understanding of how services were provided. Consequently, the directors could only rarely describe a strategy for creating systems change or articulate what they viewed to be the ideal system. Without more refined notions of how a program is to operate or what systems changes are sought, projects are likely to continue focusing their efforts on more concrete activities that may only by chance link to change within the system.

2. *Foundation leadership and direction may be critical in guiding demonstration initiatives.* In addressing emerging and ill-defined problem areas such as homelessness among families, the leadership for developing theories and strategies of intervention may need to come from a central funder or demonstration sponsor. Although there may be merit in the local generation of ideas and strategies, the experience of the Homeless Families Program highlights the positive effects of national leadership and direction by both The Robert Wood Johnson Foundation and HUD.

3. *Because case management can be an elusive intervention, careful design and quality control are needed to ensure that it is clearly defined, implemented, and measured.* Rarely has case management been studied as comprehensively as in the Homeless Families Program evaluation. Our findings illustrate how intensive case management can often be intensive in name only; the amount of contact provided to families was rarely what was expected. For greater quality control, it may be important to monitor the amount of case management actually provided, define carefully its key components such as supervision and case mix, and develop safeguards so case managers do not get spread too thin.

4. *Housing locators can be an important addition at public housing authorities and other agencies working to house homeless families, especially in areas where housing is at a premium.* The HFP experimented with a form of housing search that was seemingly helpful in finding housing for families and in working with landlords so that they would be more willing to accept the Section 8 certificate and to

house families with limited, and often troubled, housing records. In housing markets where landlords can often receive rents higher than those the Section 8 certificate allows, finding affordable housing is a formidable task. For families who have limited negotiating skills, lack transportation, and often need to bring their children with them, the task becomes almost impossible, even if they can afford the Section 8 rents. The appointment of a housing locator is worth exploring as a way to even the playing field in cities where homeless and other families have been generally unsuccessful in the housing market.

5.   *Mental health problems stemming from domestic violence, childhood abuse, and other life struggles continue to be unmet and to challenge families' abilities to remain stable unless eligibility guidelines for public mental health services are broadened.* The findings of the Homeless Families Program evaluation illustrate the multiple psychological stresses that homeless mothers face. Although many of the stresses are not unique to homeless mothers, they are compounded by the harsh realities of frequent moves, difficult and often intolerable living conditions, and a lack of resources to meet even the most basic of needs for oneself and one's children. These stresses, often pervasive and long-standing, may paralyze an individual and limit her ability to function effectively.

Welfare and other reforms suggest that many of these family stresses may continue, and even increase. There is a need for mental health services that can aid families in coping with these stresses. It is telling that six of the Homeless Families Program projects integrated mental health services into their efforts once they started to serve families; they did not believe that they could handle families' needs through case management alone. Current restrictions make it impossible to provide public mental health services to families in a timely manner unless a family member has a severe and persistent mental illness. Although intended to ensure that limited federal and state resources are directed to those truly in need and not to the "worried well," these restrictions need to be revisited in light of the increasing evidence of domestic violence and other risk factors experienced by families, homeless or otherwise.

CONCLUSION

Homeless families, especially those with multiple problems, are challenged by the reforms under way in welfare, health, and housing. The gains in residential stability achieved by the families in the Homeless

Families Program are encouraging, particularly in view of the long histories of housing instability and other life struggles they have endured. However, families' reliance on federal support for their basic needs and their lack of steady progress in employment raise questions about how long their situations will remain stable. Moreover, the HFP findings suggest an ominous situation for other families who are currently homeless, particularly those who mirror the profile of the HFP families. Since these families have consistently fallen out of the system, the only real gain they have experienced in the last five years is staying in permanent housing. The Section 8 housing subsidy, in particular, appears to have pushed the majority of families above the threshold. Few have gone beyond that, however, and most continue to lack jobs, child care, and often sufficient education. Cutbacks in welfare present a formidable challenge for these families. The lack of consistent employment among families during their stay in the HFP suggests that these families continue to remain at risk of homelessness and that, unless major changes are also provided in the employment environment, the risk increases with welfare reforms. If Section 8 reforms also limit the time Section 8 certificates can be used, a return to homelessness for many families seems inevitable.

Endnotes

1. J. Wright, *Address Unknown: The Homeless in America* (New York: Aldine de Gruyter, 1989).
2. U.S. Conference of Mayors, *The Continued Growth of Hunger, Homelessness and Poverty in America's Cities, 1986: A 25 City Survey* (Washington, D.C.: author, 1986); U. S. Conference of Mayors, *A Status Report on Hunger and Homelessness in America's Cities: 1988: A 27 City Survey* (Washington, D.C.: author, 1989); M. Burt and B. Cohen, *America's Homeless: Numbers, Characteristics, and Programs That Serve Them* (Washington, D.C.: Urban Institute Press, 1989); Wright (1989).
3. P. W. Brickner, L. K. Scharer, B. A. Conanan, M. Savarese, and B. C. Scanlan (eds.), *Under the Safety Net: The Health and Social Welfare of the Homeless in the United States* (New York: United Hospital Fund Book, Norton, 1990).
4. See J. Wright and E. Weber, *Homelessness and Health* (Washington, D.C.: McGraw-Hill Healthcare Information Center, 1987); Wright (1989); U.S. Department of Housing and Urban Development, *The 1988 National Survey of Shelters for the Homeless* (Washington, D.C.: author, 1988).

5. See H. Goldman, J. Morrissey, and S. Ridgely, "Evaluating the Robert Wood Johnson Foundation Program on Chronic Mental Illness," *Millbank Quarterly* 72 (1994), 37–47.

6. With a Section 8 housing certificate, a family pays 30 percent of its income toward rent and utilities. Most HFP Section 8s were tenant-based, allowing the family to use the subsidy for any apartment on the open market for which the landlord would accept the certificate.

7. To address these questions, the study had two major components: multiple case studies involving the nine project areas and three comparison areas (the HFP sites were Atlanta, Baltimore, Metro Denver, Houston, Nashville, Oakland, Portland, San Francisco, and Seattle; comparison sites were San Jose/Santa Clara County, Cincinnati, and Pittsburgh) where the project was not in place, and the collection of extensive family-level data. The case studies, designed to understand the systems within each site and how they changed over time, included review of key documents; conducting a series of on-site interviews, with a variety of individual interviews, and both family and staff focus groups; conducting observations and tours of project and system services and other activities; and making telephone follow-up interviews.

   Data on families were collected through a uniform data-collection system (or management information system) designed by the evaluation team in concert with the projects. The data were collected by each family's case manager, who tracked the family from the time they entered the program until they either voluntarily left or were terminated from services. The data system provides an opportunity to learn more about the needs and the characteristics of the population of homeless families served by the program, and it assesses the implementation of the project by tracking each family's participation in the service system.

   In addition, a comprehensive assessment, administered by trained interviewers, was completed with mothers in HFP families who remained in services-enriched housing four months or longer. The assessment was designed to learn more about families who had had a minimum level of participation in the program. Of the 1,207 families eligible for family assessment, 781 completed the interview (65 percent). Information was also routinely collected from the public housing authorities on the residential status of all families after they left the program.

8. For results from other studies of homeless families, see P. Rossi, "Troubling Families: Family Homelessness in America," *American Behavioral Scientist,* 37 (1994), 342–395. For information on welfare recipients, see M. J. Bane

and D. Ellwood, *Welfare Realities: From Rhetoric to Reform* (Cambridge, Mass.: Harvard University Press, 1994).

9. Data on services are restricted to those families on whom we have a reasonably high percentage of the monthly case management contact data (80 percent or better). Across the nine sites, sufficient data were available on 75 percent of the HFP families; in five sites, data were available on 80–90 percent. Thus, the data are likely to be less representative of the entire service population, especially in some sites where the percentage is lower.

10. Because we measured the receipt of services as a case manager reporting that the mother received the service at least one time while she was in the program, it is likely that this longer time period inflates the level of receipt to some degree (in the sense that the intake figures generally consider a point in time).

11. These results, obtained through logistic regressions, should be used cautiously because of the relatively low incidence of reporting current severe violence, as well as the low incidence of residential instability.

12. The exit data are based on all families who exit (86 percent) from the HFP program. Several qualifications need to be considered when examining these numbers. First, the cited percentage working is the most conservative estimate, based on the total number of primary parents on whom exit data are obtained, including data on those whose working status is unknown (22 percent of the total). When working status is computed just on those families for whom this information is known at exit, the percentage working increases to 26 percent.

13. For more information, see D. Rog et al., "Case Management in Practice: Lessons from the Evaluation of the RAJ/HUD Homeless Families Program," *Journal of Prevention and Intervention in the Community* (forthcoming).

14. As with the services data, case management contacts are limited to families for whom 80 percent or more of the data are available. The same issues of representativeness of these data apply.

~~ The National Health and Social Life Survey

Public Health Findings and Their Implications

Robert T. Michael

Editors' Introduction

A difficult but important role for foundations is tackling issues involving important social concerns that are too controversial for the government to fund. In the 1980s, one such concern was sexual behavior and its relationship to public and individual health. The HIV epidemic was emerging, but knowledge of sexual practices influencing the transmission of this and other sexually transmitted diseases was inadequate to shape public health responses.

Despite general agreement among health specialists about the importance of obtaining this information, the government was reluctant to support research that asked people about their private sexual behavior. Although the National Institute of Child Health and Human Development (NICHD) had originally requested a national survey of sexual behavior, the idea was killed when it became known by other parts of the federal government. After that happened, a consortium of foundations stepped forward to fund it. As it turned out, the study engendered little controversy, and the anticipated concerns about respondents' reactions never materialized; rather, Americans were incredibly cooperative.

Chapter Eleven describes the experience of fielding the survey and discusses its key public health findings. The knowledge gained from this project exceeded all expectations, and the findings gained widespread attention from the general public as well as public health experts, from cover stories in weekly newsmagazines to the many articles in academic journals.

This project exemplifies a number of the Foundation's goals and strategies. First, it involved collaboration with other funders; cross-foundation funding generally strengthens projects and aids in dissemination. Second, reports from the survey have been directed at diverse audiences, ranging from researchers and public health officials to the public. Two distinct books that read as if they could never have come from the same study were published: one for the general public and one for experts and researchers who specialize in social, behavioral, and cultural aspects of sexual behavior. Finally, in this project the Foundation complemented its action-oriented investment—in a series of demonstration projects about how to improve preventive and acute services related to HIV illness—with a research investment to better understand the roots of the problem. Combining research, which can make a contribution in the long run, with demonstration and service investments, which provide more immediate contributions to resolving a social problem, has been important to the Foundation.

Robert T. Michael, the author of this chapter on sexual behavior, is Eliakim Hastings Moore Distinguished Service Professor, the Irving B. Harris Graduate School of Public Policy Studies at the University of Chicago, and a leading survey researcher. With Edward O. Laumann and John H. Gagnon, he coordinated the study. He has made a series of important contributions to the literature on sexual behavior.

T he discovery of HIV in the early 1980s caught the nation ill-prepared. There was far too little accumulated knowledge about retrovirology and far too little continuing research. In 1986, the National Institutes of Health (NIH) said publicly that scientists were unlikely to cure or prevent AIDS through biomedical research until sometime after the beginning of the 1990s. Unfortunately, even that assessment was too optimistic.

Society was at least as ill-prepared as science, with too little knowledge and too little continuing social science research about the primary means of transmitting HIV: sexual relations. In the late 1980s, the high-priority need in the social sciences was data on the sexual behavior of the general public, on a national basis and not exclusively focused on any particular sexual practice. The Institute of Medicine took this position in 1986, and it was endorsed by the report of the Presidential Commission on the HIV Epidemic in 1988 and by commissions and panels of National Academy of Sciences/National Research Council in 1989 and by the General Accounting Office report on AIDS forecasting, also in 1989.[1] Many public and private statements by medical and social science scholars and administrators and by the chief executive officers of pharmaceutical companies mirrored that view.[2]

By the late 1980s, it was understood that HIV was transmitted from one person to another by three means—sexual contact, sharing needles in intravenous drug usage, and blood transfusions—and the most common of these methods was sexual contact. The *HIV/AIDS Surveillance Report*, issued by the Centers for Disease Control (CDC) in January 1990, reported on the cumulative AIDS cases in the United States through December 1989. There were 115,786 adult cases of AIDS, about two-thirds of which were attributed to sexual contact, about one-quarter to intravenous drug usage, and only 2 percent to blood transfusions, with the remainder undetermined or by multiple means.[3] While public health officials understood that sexual behavior was the major route by which the virus was spread, they also recognized that they did not know very much about the incidence of various sexual activities that facilitated transmission.

The 1989 report by the National Research Council, *AIDS: Sexual Behavior and Intravenous Drug Use,* makes clear why the information about sexual behavior was needed:

Estimating future demands on hospitals and other public health services requires reliable models of HIV transmission dynamics. Such
epidemiological models . . . can also help in assessing the relative effectiveness of different kinds of behavioral change and guiding the development of effective public health education.

Data needs are driven by immediately relevant questions of disease
transmission, progress, and control. The resulting intellectual strategy
is to design new research looking for the "facts about sex" in order to
answer these questions.

The report goes on to argue for understanding the social context
of the sexual behavior:

To understand the motives, development, and varieties of human sexual behavior, it is crucial to understand the systems of meaning and
action—the cultural context—in which the "facts of sex" are embedded. The facts remain the same, but understanding may differ. Different understandings in turn may have important consequences for
designing effective educational efforts to encourage self-protective
behaviors.[4]

By 1987, the leadership at NIH was encouraging and funding relevant social science research. By mid–1988, the CDC was urging the
collection, before the 1980s came to an end, of baseline information
about sexual behavior of the general population. Because of the political ambivalence about the survey research, however, little more was
known about sexual behavior as it related to the transmission of HIV
by, say, 1991, than had been known a decade earlier, when HIV was
beginning to surface. Much of the little additional insight was derived
from research that was not publicly funded.[5]

This research project's experience with the federal government was
protracted and complex, reflecting that political ambivalence. The
history from 1987 through 1991 was typical of the experience of
other survey projects that attempted to respond to the need to know
more about sexual practices as they relate to the transmission of HIV.
The government's stance might best be described as inconsistent or
even schizophrenic. The less political and more scientific the entity
(at one extreme, for instance, the peer review system at NIH), the
more supportive the attitude toward these research efforts; conversely,
the more political and less scientific the entity (at the other extreme,
deliberation on Capitol Hill), the less supportive attitudes were.

Specifically, our project began in response to a National Institute of Child Health and Human Development request for proposals in July 1987, seeking advice about the design of a national survey of adult sexual behavior as related to reproductive health and sexually transmitted diseases, including HIV. My colleagues, Edward O. Laumann and John H. Gagnon, and I responded to the NICHD request through the National Opinion Research Center, or NORC, at the University of Chicago. We won the competition to design that survey, and before our one-year effort was completed in 1988, NICHD and CDC requested another proposal to put that design into practice in order to produce baseline data before the end of the 1980s about adult sexual behavior in the United States. Our team competed for that contract as well and won it. The design of the survey was completed by the autumn of 1988.

As required of any survey of Americans done under contract with the federal government, we submitted routine documents and materials for clearance from the Office of Management and Budget (OMB), expecting to begin conducting the survey in January 1989. In brief, OMB never gave us the necessary clearance. Instead, it referred the question of whether our survey of adult sexual behavior could or should be done to the top levels of the Department of Health and Human Services; the survey subsequently became an issue on Capitol Hill. Through stages and complexities that are described elsewhere,[6] we were finally informed in late summer 1991 that the federal government was not willing to approve a study of adult sexual behavior, even though it had initially requested one. At that juncture, Laumann, Gagnon, and I received support for our project from The Robert Wood Johnson Foundation.

The contrast between the federal government's ambivalence and the position of the Foundation is clearly seen by the project's title in the two settings. Essentially the same project was titled by the NICHD's request for proposals as "Social and Behavioral Aspects of Health and Fertility-Related Behavior." Our grant application to the Foundation, in April 1991, was titled "Sexual Behavior and Its Relation to the Health of the American Population"—a decidedly more direct and informative title.

The two-year project undertaken with Foundation support involved a national survey of the sexual behavior of adults age eighteen to fifty-nine, selected from a stratified random sample of households and interviewed over the period February to September 1992.

Immediately before and during the field period of the survey, additional funding was secured from the Henry J. Kaiser Family Foundation, the Rockefeller Foundation, the Andrew Mellon Foundation, the John D. and Catherine T. MacArthur Foundation, the New York Community Trust, and the American Foundation for AIDS Research, and subsequently, for data analysis, from the Ford Foundation. Thus, the project has had wide and enthusiastic support from the American foundation community.

The survey was done by face-to-face interview, typically in the respondent's home. It was conducted by about 220 NORC interviewers who had undergone an intensive, three-day training session on the questionnaire. The survey asked basic demographic, economic, and social background facts about the respondent, including histories of all marriages, cohabitational intervals, and conceptions and their outcomes. It asked about sexual behavior over the past year, then in greater detail regarding the respondent's most recent sexual event, and then more generally about sexual behavior over the whole lifetime. Information was also obtained about childhood sexual experiences, adolescent sexual experiences, sexual victimization, sexual health including both lifetime and past-year sexually transmitted infections, sexual dysfunctions, and finally about sexual attitudes and opinions.

The cooperation of 3,432 adults in the survey was outstanding. The survey had an exceptionally high response rate: 79 percent, or nearly four of every five randomly selected men and women from coast to coast, were willing to cooperate by responding to questions about their intimate sexual behavior. Care was taken in the interview to establish an environment of privacy, safety, and trust with the respondents; a strong public health motivation was used to encourage honesty and accuracy. Also, much care was taken to achieve the right balance of scope and detail about the sexual behavior so that respondents could and would want to provide accurate answers. Subject to the limits of personal interviewing on any topic, these efforts seemed to be very effective. From internal consistency checks and from external validation of much of the information collected, it appears that this data set is of exceptionally high quality. Two books report the initial findings from the survey,[7] one intended for a general audience, the other for a scientific audience. The public-use dataset, known as the National Health and Social Life Survey (NHSLS), was put in the public domain through Sociometrics, Inc., in December 1994. (It is also available through the Interuniversity Consortium for Political and Social Research, or ICPSR, of the University of Michigan.)

Fortunately, this survey has by now become one of several high-quality datasets addressing sexual behavior and sexual health.[8] So despite the initial political difficulties, there have been successful efforts to collect survey data about sexual behavior, and the American population has been cooperative and forthcoming.

PUBLIC HEALTH FINDINGS

There were six major public health findings from the NHSLS. The first three pertain to traditional issues about the spread of infectious diseases: how widespread they are, what their primary risk factors are, and why these factors represent such high risks. The other three are facts about how people behave, since their behavior has implications for our understanding of the spread of these diseases. These facts include evidence of purposive, strategic behavior on the part of individuals to avoid diseases; evidence of the social context in which sexual partnering occurs; and evidence that adult sexual behavior can be determined from surveys using proper scientific sampling. All six of these findings should be considered part of the nation's public health agenda.

1.   *Most sexually transmitted infections are contracted by young adults (under age thirty), and these infections flourish in that relatively small segment of the population.* Most data on sexually transmitted infections, or STIs, come from clinic-based studies or from national registry data such as the CDC's surveillance reports. Neither of these can provide information about the proportion of the population that has, or has ever had, one of these diseases. The counts of specific infections are not usually identified by patient, so we cannot know from these sources how many different diseases one person may have had, or how often one person may have been diagnosed with the same disease. Thus, one cannot estimate the prevalence of the disease in the population at large or in population subgroups, but for epidemiological projections this is the information that it is important to know.

Surveys that ask about some of these infections in general population samples typically do not obtain very much information about the sexual practices of the respondents, so even when we know how many new cases there are, or what proportion of the population is infected, we still do not have the information to permit an assessment of behavioral risk. The National Health and Social Life Survey data do yield estimates of both the incidence and the prevalence of sexually transmitted infections, and those two factors constitute the first two findings described here.

The NHSLS asked specifically about nine infections: gonorrhea, syphilis, genital herpes, chlamydia, genital warts, hepatitis, HIV/AIDS, and pelvic inflammatory disease (PID, women only) and nongonococcal urethritis (NGU, men only).[9] The question asked if the respondent had ever been told by a doctor that he or she had one of these infections; each infection was asked about specifically and separately. If the answer was yes, the respondent was asked how many times and whether that diagnosis had been within the past twelve months, where he or she went for treatment, and which sex partner the respondent thought may have given him or her the disease. For much of the analysis we have done to date, we have considered the five bacterial infections together (gonorrhea, syphilis, chlamydia, NGU, and PID) and similarly the four viral infections (Hepatitis B, genital warts, genital herpes, and HIV). The former are relatively easy to cure with antibiotics in the early stages soon after presentation, while the latter are incurable and in some cases recurring, so the health risks differ for these two types of infection.

Overall, 16.9 percent of adults age eighteen to fifty-nine report that they have had a diagnosed sexually transmitted infection sometime in their life, and 1.6 percent say they have had that diagnosis within the past twelve months. The lifetime rates are similar for men and women overall, although the men report higher rates of bacterial infections (12.1 percent for men, 10.6 percent for women), primarily gonorrhea, while women report higher rates of viral infections (9.0 percent for women, 5.4 percent for men). The rate of infection reported in our survey for the past twelve-month period is 1.6 percent overall, with 1.0 percent for bacterial infections and 0.6 percent for viral infections.

By age, the lifetime rates reach 17–19 percent by the late twenties and remain at about that level up to age fifty; they are then lower (about 11 percent) for those who are over fifty. The rates of those who report having a diagnosed STI within the past year are highest among young adults: 4.5 percent of people between eighteen and twenty-one compared with less than 1 percent for any age group over thirty. Clearly, it is the young adults who acquire and transmit most STIs. If one in twenty-two young adults has an STI within a year (that is, 4.5

percent), the risk is substantial that someone who has several sex partners selected from that pool is exposed to disease. With rates of infection as high as one in two, as is estimated for gonorrhea, the likelihood of contracting a disease is indeed considerable for someone with multiple sex partners in a year.[10]

The information about STIs collected in our study is retrospective, collected at a point in time. With information of this nature, one cannot distinguish a "cohort effect" (a difference for those born at one time from those born at another time, such as the population born at the peak of the baby boom, in 1957) from an "age effect" (a difference that all experience at a particular age, such as puberty). Thus, we cannot tell if the younger generation will continue to acquire sexually transmitted infections at a high rate as they age or will experience a decline in the rates of contracting diseases as they age beyond thirty. The data clearly show, however, that most STIs have been contracted by young adults, and it is in that relatively small portion of the whole population that these infections flourish.

2.   *The number of sex partners is the single most important risk factor for getting a sexually transmitted infection.* In descriptive tables of who gets STIs, age is often shown as an important demographic factor. But in our statistical work we are able to look for the basic reasons that some people do and others do not get STIs and that statistical analysis of STI risks shows that age per se is not a risk factor. We have studied the partial effects of age, gender, race/ethnicity, education level, marital status, number of sex partners, and exposure to specific sex practices such as group sex, anal sex, and paid sex. Overwhelmingly the most important single factor, for both bacterial and viral STIs, is the number of sexual partners. In fact, age is not statistically significant once these more directly influential factors are controlled. Similarly, marital status and education level show no relationship with either type of infection.

Those with more than ten lifetime sexual partners are estimated to be twenty times as likely to have contracted an STI as those with one lifetime partner. Those with five to ten lifetime partners are nine times as likely to have acquired a bacterial infection and five times as likely to have acquired a viral infection; those with two to four lifetime partners are about two and a half times as likely to have had an STI as those with one lifetime partner. It is this factor—the number of partners—that dramatically dominates the risk of a sexually transmitted disease. Clearly, the reason young adults acquire these diseases has nothing directly to do with their age per se; the behavior that creates the risk is having many sex partners, and it is primarily young, unmarried adults who engage in that behavior.

Men face a much lower risk of contracting these diseases than women. Controlled for number of partners, men have only about 40 percent the risk women face of getting a bacterial infection and only about 30 percent the risk women face of getting a viral infection, according to our survey results. That fact conforms with what is known about the infectivity of many of these diseases: they are more easily transmitted from a male to a female than vice versa. Thus, we should expect to find the evidence that we do: when the number of sex partners is held constant, the risks of an STI are substantially higher for women.

Blacks report fourfold higher rates of bacterial infection, mostly gonorrhea, other factors held constant, while they have rates of viral infection only about half as high as whites. The explanation for this is clear, we think. Our study found dramatic evidence of the social embeddedness of the selection of sex partners, meaning that blacks tend to have sex with other blacks and whites tend to have sex with other whites.[11] If a disease is prevalent within a social group, especially one with a high infectivity, such as gonorrhea, it is likely to be readily transmitted within that group, but not necessarily readily spread to other groups if few from the first group have sex with members of the second group. The concentration of gonorrhea within the young black community probably reflects this phenomenon. That concentration may also be influenced by the fact that blacks and whites may go to different sorts of institutions for medical treatment. What is more, public clinics and private physicians may not approach an infection in the same way. Both tests and treatment may differ, and so may the reports to patients and to public health officials.

The statistical analyses also suggest that those who have ever engaged in anal sex have somewhat higher rates of viral infection, while those who have been paid for sex are twice as likely to have had a bacterial infection. Those who have had one type of STI (bacterial or viral) are about twice as likely to have also had the other type as well.

3.   *The reason that someone with many partners has a high risk of an STI is that those other partners also have many partners, often concurrently. Those who have many partners will not know all of their*

partners well and are unlikely to have as strong a personal concern about them as someone who has few sexual partners, or just one partner. We have attempted to go behind the strong evidence in the survey data that the number of sex partners is the overwhelmingly dominant factor associated with the risk of disease, and look at two aspects of the "partner risk." The majority of sexually active adults do not acquire new sex partners in any given year and are exposed to relatively low risks of contracting sexually transmitted disease. Others—about 20 percent of our sample of adults—do acquire a new partner within the year. We focused on two dimensions of sexual partnerships, the *familiarity* of the respondent and his or her partner, and the *sexual exclusivity* of their relationship, as assessed by the respondent.

We contend that greater familiarity with a sex partner is likely to be associated with greater comfort in discussing sexual histories and risk-reducing strategies, with greater information about the disease status of that partner, with greater caring and concern, and thus greater motivation to protect the partner from disease. Our measures of familiarity include having a new partner within the past twelve months, having a one-time sex partner, having sex with the person for less than a two-month interval, knowing the person less than two days or less than one month prior to first having sex with him or her, and self-descriptions of the relationship as casual sex or a pick-up partner.

We measure sexual exclusivity by several variables, including the number of sex partners the respondent reported his or her partner to have had within the past year, whether that partner was involved with another person at the onset of their sexual relationship, whether that partner continued to have sex with others (distinguishing serial and concurrent partnerships, which have very different implications for disease transmission), whether the partnership involved an expectation of sexual exclusivity, and whether the partnership involved explicit payment for sex.

The evidence shows dramatically that those who have one sex partner tend to have long-term associations and sexual exclusivity with that partner and thus face very little risk of an STI. In contrast, those who have many sex partners face a higher risk of an STI. They report that their partners also have many other partners, tend to be not as well known to the respondent, and have relatively little familiarity or commitment or personal concern.

These differences, then, translate into a much higher risk of disease and explain why the number of sex partners is such a powerful indicator of that risk. When we investigate the relationships between one or another of these measures of familiarity or exclusivity and STIs, we find that the rates of disease are typically three or so times as high for adults who have partners with these risky attributes. For example, the rates of being diagnosed with an STI within the past twelve months are 3.6 times as high for an adult who has any new sex partner within that time interval; 4.3 times as high for one who has any one-time sex partner within that time interval; and 2.2 times as high for one who had a partner with whom monogamy was not expected. Taking several of these partner attributes in combination, 0.8 percent of those whose partners have none of the several measured risky attributes reported an STI within the past twelve months; 2.2 percent of those with one of those attributes reported an STI; and as many as 5.5 percent of those whose partners totaled at least four of those attributes reported an STI within the past twelve months. If that 5.5 percent per annum were the exposure faced by a person for several consecutive years, the accumulated probability of contracting an STI would become quite high, and that may well be the experience for a substantial number of young adults.

4.   *People at high risk of getting a sexually transmitted disease are changing their sexual behavior.* One of the more optimistic findings from the analysis of the survey data is evidence of effective, purposive, strategic behavior in response to the risks of getting an STI. One of those behaviors is the use of condoms. Condom use is highly situational: only 8 percent of married adults in the survey reported that they always used a condom in the past twelve months with their spouse, while 11 percent of those who had a cohabitational partner did so, and 29 percent of those who were neither married nor living with their primary sex partner always used a condom in the past twelve months.

Measured by whether they used a condom the most recent time they had sex, 14 percent of those with one partner within the past twelve months did so, 26 percent of those with two partners did so, 36 percent of those with three partners did so, 40 percent of those with four partners did so, but only 30 percent of those with five or more partners did so. Clearly, those who face higher risk of disease because they have more partners do respond by using condoms more consistently. The levels of use, however, are not sufficiently high to justify any less effort at promoting safer sex by public health officials, and there is disquieting evidence here of a small core of high-risk individuals who are not exercising preventive behavior.

As many as 30 percent of the adult population report making some change in their sexual behavior because of AIDS. There are many strategies that can be effective in reducing the risk of contracting HIV, and most of these are effective at preventing other, more prevalent STIs as well. Of that 30 percent of the survey respondents who report a change in their behavior, many report more than one change, and in terms of the more common changes that are reported, roughly one-quarter report each of the following: using condoms more frequently, now having only one partner, and selecting their partners more carefully or getting to know their partners better before having sex. Also, 11 percent report having reduced their number of partners, and 11 percent report that they now abstain from sex altogether.

It is encouraging to find that those most likely to report risk-reducing strategies are precisely those who have previously engaged in the riskiest sex practices. For example, 78 percent of those with eleven to twenty partners in the past five years report making a change in their sexual behavior, while only 12 percent of those with one partner in the past five years report any change in behavior. Specifically, if we compare those with eleven or more partners within the past five years to those with four or fewer partners, the former are nearly five times as likely to report reducing their number of sex partners, twice as likely to report selecting their partners more carefully now, and three times as likely to report using condoms more now.

5.   *Most people have sex with others who are similar to themselves in terms of age, education, race, and most other social attributes. This dramatically inhibits the spread of STIs among the population at large.* Sexual partnerships are deeply embedded in social structures. For our understanding of the transmission of disease, perhaps the most important long-term finding from the National Health and Social Life Survey data is that sexual partners are overwhelmingly similar in their demographic and social characteristics. They are remarkably similar in age, in race (African American or white) and in ethnicity (Hispanic or non-Hispanic), in education, and in religion. The survey inquired about secondary sex partners and one-time partners as well as the respondent's "primary" or regular sex partner. While we expected that primary sex partners would be similar in these demographic dimensions, we thought that the casual or one-time or other secondary part-

ners would perhaps be much more different and would constitute a big threat in terms of transmitting a disease from one group in society to another. So we attempted in many ways to determine if those in one social stratum frequently or infrequently had sex with someone from another social stratum. We did find some who have sex with others from different social groups, and who do therefore provide a bridge across which diseases might travel, but they are few and their pattern of bridging is infrequent.

It has been well known that married couples are typically similar in these social characteristics, but we find that even very short-term, noncohabiting pairs are remarkably similar: 91 percent of these short-term pairs are of the same race or ethnicity, 87 percent are of the same educational level, and 60 percent are from similar religious faiths.

Another way of thinking about the issue of the spread of a sexually transmitted infection is to think of the social network of individuals in a community. Imagine a randomly selected individual and think about how many others in that community that one person is connected to. If the definition of "connected" is that that individual knows another person or that the two know someone in common, then their social network is likely to be very densely connected. But if the definition of "connected" is that they have sex with each other, or have sex with someone in common, then the evidence from the survey data suggests that their sexual network is very sparsely connected. Moreover, that sexual network is effectively partitioned by social characteristics such as race or ethnicity, education, age, and religion. This implies that the social organization of sex partnering in our communities makes it rather unlikely that a sexually transmitted infection will spread throughout that community. However, for those infections that pass from an infected person to another quite easily—such as gonorrhea—even a few bridge people in the community can carry the infection across social boundaries. In the case of a disease that does not spread easily, the social organization of sex partnering makes it unlikely that the disease will spread. Fortunately, HIV is a virus that has a very low infectivity, of about one in five hundred, so it is not a likely candidate for easy transmission from one social network to another.

6.   *Under the proper circumstances, adults in the United States will cooperate in a scientific survey about their sexual behavior.* It has been dogma in our nation, at least since the time of its pronouncement by

the sex researcher Alfred Kinsey in 1948,[12] that a randomly selected sample of Americans would not cooperate in a social scientific survey about their sexual behavior. That dogma encouraged Kinsey and many others since that time to accept unscientific sampling as the only feasible way to study sexual behavior by survey. Consequently, when AIDS appeared and the need arose to understand the likely route and speed of its transmission through sexual activity in the population, public health officials were ill-prepared. The National Health and Social Life Survey has shown that dogma to be incorrect. It is a major finding of this project that Americans can be interviewed in scientifically appropriate ways about their sexual behavior. They cooperate in such a survey. They provide the necessary information when they are assured of confidentiality and when they are convinced of the merit and appropriateness of the survey's purpose. Unfortunately, learning about HIV provides that purpose.

We cannot know now if the cooperativeness experienced in the survey would have been the same twenty or forty years before, when HIV was unknown. The assertion by Kinsey in his day, and by many others as recently as the late 1980s, that a survey could not be done was simply accepted without good evidence. An enduring and important public health finding of this project is that that assertion is wrong.

IMPLICATIONS FOR PUBLIC HEALTH POLICY

With as many as one in six adults under age sixty reporting that they have had a sexually transmitted disease sometime in their lifetime, and with more than one in twenty young adults age eighteen to twenty-four reporting that they have had one of these diseases within the past twelve months, there is no basis for complacency in our public health policy toward STIs. There is strong evidence that the risks of these diseases are not uniformly spread among the population, so it would seem prudent to target both preventive educational efforts and remedial medical attention upon the young, single adults where those diseases are most prevalent.

The risk factors for STIs are well known. The National Health and Social Life Survey contributes strong evidence that the number of sex partners is *the* key risk factor. Demographic or social characteristics including age, education, religion, race or ethnicity, and religion play a role only to the degree that they affect the number of sex partners.

Those with ten or more lifetime sex partners are twenty times as likely to have an STI as those with one lifetime partner. That fact should be made part of the public health message and should be aimed at young single adults, since it is they who have the most partners.

The survey also indicates that certain population subgroups can and do develop high prevalences for some diseases. Since sex partnerships are so systematically drawn from groups of similar individuals, diseases can be found in one group with very little implication for the likelihood of finding them in some other group. The evidence in the survey of gonorrhea among young blacks is but an example. It could be as true of an infectious disease in a college-based population or any other group that happens to have high rates of sexual interaction.

While the proportion of adults who report having as many as five sexual partners in a year is no higher than 3.2 percent, and those with more than twenty partners within the past five years is no higher than 1.7 percent, for example, it must be stressed that these are not small numbers of people. One percent of the adult population age eighteen to fifty-nine is about 1.5 million people.

The survey also helps understand why having many sex partners is associated with so much higher risk of STIs. It is not the case that a man with five partners in a year has only five times as much risk as the man with one partner. That would be the case if all five of those partners were similar in their risky attributes. But that is not what is found: the more partners one has, the more likely they are to have risky attributes, such as being much less well known to the subject and having had several other partners themselves. The familiarity with, and the exclusivity of, partners declines as the number of partners increases, and that raises the risks of disease. The implication for public health policy would appear to be to encourage young adults to be more selective and strategic in their choice of partners and to be strategic in minimizing concurrent partnerships, as well as adopting risk-reducing practices in their sexual repertoire.

The survey suggests that much strategic behavior is undertaken to reduce the risks of disease in sexual relationships. Condom usage is higher where the risks are greater. Of the 30 percent of adults who say they have changed their behavior because of AIDS, those whose behavior puts them most at risk are indeed those who have changed their behavior, and in general the nature of the changes has been broadly appropriate. Nonetheless, of those with more than ten sex partners within the past five years, nearly one-third report having made no change in their sexual behavior because of risks of disease. Here, again, public education and persuasion effort are called for.

The survey data emphasize the similarity of sex partners in terms of their social characteristics, and this has implications for the risks of spread of disease. This important finding has both an optimistic and a pessimistic implication. It implies that a disease does not so easily spread through the entire population as it might if those social barriers to its transmission were less severe. On the other hand, the social embeddedness of sexual life makes it more likely that one disease or another may be considered "their" problem, not "ours," which could undermine a public commitment to addressing the risks with effective education, medical care access, and research funding.

There have now been several other scientifically sound surveys of sexual behavior, and there should be more. The National Health and Social Life Survey, in its ninety-minute interview, began a process of inquiry that deserves continued funding and research commitment. It has been the social and public health policy in the United States to settle for inadequate information and understanding about sexual behavior, as if, because it is private behavior, it is acceptable not to know very much about it. But public health and social policy require that Americans reach collective decisions about many aspects of sexual life, from accessing contraceptives to accessing pornography. Americans have a need and a right to know about the prevalence of specific sexually transmitted diseases and their various rates of infectivity, about how common various sexual practices are and about how common specific sexual dysfunctions are, and about how many adults do or do not engage in homosexual behavior, for example.

The survey has only begun to provide answers to these questions; it should be a beginning of a growing inquiry into sexual behavior and practices and their consequences. My colleagues and I hope that its legacy is to have destroyed the myth that we cannot successfully survey Americans about their sexual behavior.

Endnotes

1. Institute of Medicine, *Confronting AIDS: Directions for Public Health, Health Care and Research* (1986); *Report of the Presidential Commission on the Human Immunodeficiency Virus Epidemic* (1988); National Research Council, *AIDS: Sexual Behavior and Intravenous Drug Use* (1989); U.S.

Congress General Accounting Office Report, *AIDS Forecasting: Undercount of Cases and Lack of Key Data Weaken Existing Estimate* (1989).

2. Ted Cooper, Upjohn Co.; Florence Haseltine, director, CPR, NICHD; Don des Jarlais, coordinator for AIDS Research New York State Division of Substance Abuse Services and Drug Research; Philip Lee, School of Medicine, UCSF; Jane Menken, professor of sociology, University of Pennsylvania and chair, NRC Committee on AIDS Research and the Behavioral, Social, and Statistical Sciences; June Osborn, dean of School of Public Health, University of Michigan and chair, National Commission on AIDS; Samuel Their, president, Institute of Medicine; Ronald Wilson, AIDS coordinator, National Center for Health Statistics.

3. Centers for Disease Control, *HIV/AIDS Surveillance Report* (Jan. 1990), p. 9.

4. C. F. Turner, H. G. Miller, and L. E. Moses (eds.), *AIDS: Sexual Behavior and Intravenous Drug Use* (Washington D.C.: National Academy Press, 1989), p. 78.

5. For example, see *MMWR* 37(37) (Sept. 23, 1988), 565–568.

6. E. O. Laumann, R. T. Michael, and J. H. Gagnon, "A Political History of the National Sex Survey of Adults," *Family Planning Perspectives* 26(1) (Jan.–Feb. 1994), 34–38.

7. R. T. Michael, J. H. Gagnon, E. O. Laumann, and G. Kolata, *Sex in America* (New York: Little, Brown, 1994); and E. O. Laumann, J. H. Gagnon, R. T. Michael, and S. Michaels, *The Social Organization of Sexuality* (Chicago: University of Chicago Press, 1994).

8. Other national in-person surveys and their principal investigators include the National Survey of Adolescent Males, done in 1988 and 1990–1991 by F. L. Sonenstein and her colleagues; the National Surveys of Men and of Women, done in 1991 under the leadership of K. Tanfer; the twenty-thousand–person Survey of Adolescent Health in 1995 under J. R. Udry's direction; the National Survey of Family Growth conducted through NCHS in 1988 (Cycle IV) and 1990 (Cycle IV phone reinterview) with data for women age 15–44 on contraception, number of partners, AIDS-related behavior and STIs; and for annual time series (1988–1996) on a few sexual behaviors, the General Social Survey, led by J. A. Davis and T. Smith. Additionally, a national telephone survey of individuals age 18–75, the National AIDS Behavioral Surveys in 1990–91 (wave 1) and 1992 (wave 2), led by J. A. Cataria has also yielded important results. There have also been a number of local area, or state-level surveys, and many others that focus on one or another specific high-risk group or high-risk behavior.

9. A tenth infection, vaginitis, was not analyzed since some common forms can be contracted nonsexually (for example, from yeast infections)

although other forms of this generic are among the most common reported by CDC (for example, trichomoniasis).

10. The likelihood of contracting a disease from a simple act of intercourse with a randomly selected partner is the product $P \times I$, where P is the disease's prevalence in the population from which that partner was selected, and I is the disease's rate of infectivity or transmissibility. This risk is discussed in detail in chapter eleven of Laumann, Gagnon, Michael, and Michaels (1994).

11. For example, 82 percent of black men have black women as their sex partners, and 97 percent of black women have black men as their sex partners; of unmarried white men, 94 percent have white women as their sex partners, and 90 percent of single white women have white men as their partners. These figures are reported in Michael, Gagnon, Laumann, and Kolata (1994), p. 46.

12. Kinsey's colorful statement was: "Neither is it feasible to stand on a street corner, tap every tenth individual on the shoulder, and command him to contribute a full and frankly honest sex history. Theoretically less satisfactory but more practical means of sampling human material must be accepted as the best that can be done." A. C. Kinsey, W. B. Pomeroy, and C. E. Martin, *Sexual Behavior in the Human Male* (Philadelphia: Saunders, 1948), p. 93.

Ironically, Kinsey also reports his "amazement at their [his respondents'] willingness to help" by agreeing to be interviewed (p. 36). He suggests the motive often is altruism: "In answer to our request for her history, the little, gray-haired women at the cabin door, out on the Western plain, epitomized what we have heard now from hundreds of people: 'Of all things—! In all my years I have never had such a question put to me! But—if my experience will help, I'll give it to you.' This, in many forms . . . is the expression of the altruistic bent . . . which has been the chief motive leading people to cooperate in this study" (p. 36). Unfortunately, Kinsey did not follow that insight to its logical conclusion that indeed one *can* secure the cooperation of a randomly selected sample of respondents. How much more we might know today about our sexual behavior and its consequences if Kinsey had not promoted the myth that scientific sampling could not be employed in the study of human sexuality!

⟿ About the Editors

Stephen L. Isaacs, J.D., is the president of the Center for Health and Social Policy in Pelham, New York. A former professor of public health at Columbia University and founding director of its Development Law and Policy Program, Isaacs has written extensively for professional and popular audiences. His book *The Consumer's Legal Guide to Today's Health Care* was reviewed as "the single best guide to the health care system in print today"; his articles have been widely syndicated and have appeared in law reviews and health policy journals. He also provides technical assistance internationally on health law, human rights, and population policy. A graduate of Columbia Law School and Brown University, Isaacs served as vice president of International Planned Parenthood's Latin American division, practiced health law, and spent four years in Thailand as a program officer for the U.S. Agency for International Development. He serves on the Advisory Council of the National Institute of Child Health and Human Development, the Advisory Board of the Women's Rights Project of Human Rights Watch, and the board of trustees of the Royce mutual funds. He is currently completing a comprehensive analysis of the new foundations created by the conversion of nonprofit hospitals and health plans to for-profit status.

James R. Knickman, Ph.D., is vice president for research and evaluation at The Robert Wood Johnson Foundation. Prior to joining the Foundation in October 1992, he was a professor of health administration at New York University's Robert Wagner Graduate School of Public Service. He has published extensively on a range of health care issues and done research on insurance markets and health care reimbursement systems, with particular attention to long-term care services. He also has written about methods for improving health services for urban, vulnerable populations such as the homeless, the frail elderly, and individuals with HIV illness. Knickman has served on a range of state government, local government, and health care sector advisory committees and has offered consultation to numerous health sector organizations. Currently, he serves on the board of trustees of the Robert Wood Johnson University Hospital. He received his doctorate in public policy analysis from the University of Pennsylvania and did undergraduate work at Fordham University.

~~~ About the Contributors

Susan M. Allen, Ph.D., received her doctorate in sociology from Brown University. She is currently an assistant professor of medical science in the department of community health, an adjunct assistant professor in the department of sociology, and a research associate of the Population Studies and Training Center at Brown. Her research interests focus on disability, gender roles in the illness experience, and, more broadly, the home care needs and unmet needs of people living in the community with chronic health conditions and impairments. Allen is principal investigator of the longitudinal Springfield Study, which will examine the relationship between inadequate care at home and subsequent levels of acute care utilization. She is also principal investigator of a five-year FIRST award from the National Institute on Aging that examines the influence of gender roles on gender differences in health-related outcomes experienced by community-dwelling elderly couples. Finally, she is conducting a National Cancer Institute-funded randomized trial of an intervention designed to reduce stress associated with the diagnosis and treatment of breast cancer in younger women.

Robert A. Berenson, M.D., F.A.C.P., a board-certified internist, is currently medical director and a member of the board of directors of the National Capital Preferred Provider Organization, which he helped found in 1987. He is also acting CEO of the start-up National Capital Health Plan. He practiced for twelve years in a private medical group in Washington, D.C. Prior to beginning the practice in 1981, Berenson, a graduate of the Mount Sinai School of Medicine, spent three and one-half years on President Carter's White House domestic policy staff (initially as a Robert Wood Johnson Foundation Clinical Scholar), working on national health policy issues. He has been active in policy research, particularly in the areas of physician payment policy, managed care, and quality protection, and has written numerous articles on these topics for nationally recognized journals. In 1994, Berenson became national program director of the IMPACS (Improving Malpractice Prevention and Compensation Systems) program. He served as cochair of two working groups on the Clinton White House Task Force on Health Reform, one on malpractice reform, the other on the structure and function of accountable health plans. He has served as a panel member on three Institute of Medicine studies: on utilization management, priority setting for technology assessment, and priority setting for clinical practice guidelines. He is also on the editorial board of *Health Affairs.*

Marc L. Berk, Ph.D., is director of the Project HOPE Center for Health Affairs and is a recognized expert in access to care and survey design and evaluation. He received his doctorate in sociology at New York University and subsequently was senior sociologist at the Agency for Health Care Policy and Research. He has advised policy makers in both the public and private sectors about issues related to access to care. He has published extensively on access to care for vulnerable populations, the concentration of health expenditures, and cost-effective strategies for implementing household and physician surveys. In addition to his work on the Access to Care Survey, he is currently involved in the implementation of the first national probability sample of persons with HIV. He also serves as coprincipal investigator on a study of the use of health care services by undocumented immigrants.

Lawrence D. Brown, Ph.D., is professor and head of the Division of Health Policy and Management at Columbia University's School of Public Health. He received a doctorate in government from Harvard University. Before coming to Columbia in 1988, he was a senior fellow in the Brookings Institution's Governmental Studies Program and a professor at the University of Michigan's School of Public Health, where he directed the Pew Trust Health Policy Program. He is a member of the National Advisory Committee of The Robert Wood Johnson Foundation's Health Policy Research Scholars Program, the United Hospital Fund's President's Council, and the board of the Community Services Society. He serves on the Committee on Medicine and Society of the New York Academy of Medicine, as a research adviser to the Center for Studying Health Systems Change, and on the editorial board of *Medical Care Research and Review.* From 1984 to 1989, he was editor of the *Journal of Health Politics, Policy, and Law.* Brown is author of *Politics and Health Care Organization: HMOs as Federal Policy* and various monographs and articles. He writes on competitive and regulatory issues in health, on the politics of state and national strategies to achieve affordable universal coverage, and on the uses of policy analysis in the policy process.

Joel C. Cantor, Sc.D., is director of the research division of the United Hospital Fund of New York. He also serves as a research associate professor at New York University's Robert F. Wagner Graduate School of Public Service. His current work includes a study of the transition to Medicaid managed care in New York, research on policies to address the problem of the uninsured, and an evaluation of The Robert Wood Johnson Foundation Minority Medical Education Program. Prior to joining the staff of the United Hospital Fund, he served as the director of evaluation research at The Robert Wood Johnson Foundation, where among other responsibilities he developed programs in the area of medical malpractice. Cantor presently serves on the national advisory committee of the Foundation's Improving Malpractice Prevention and Compensation Systems program. In 1988, he received his doctorate in health policy and management from The Johns Hopkins School of Hygiene and Public Health, and in 1996 he was elected a fellow of the Association for Health Services Research.

Gordon H. DeFriese, Ph.D., holds appointments as professor of social medicine, epidemiology, and health policy and administration at the University of North Carolina at Chapel Hill, where he has served as the director of the University's Cecil G. Sheps Center for Health Services Research since 1973. In 1986, he became codirector of The Robert Wood Johnson Foundation's Clinical Scholars Program, cosponsored by the UNC-CH School of Medicine and the Sheps Center. His personal research interests include primary health care, rural health services, health services utilization behavior, child health services, dental care, medical technology assessment, medical self-care, health and aging, cost-effectiveness and cost-benefit analysis, medical specialization, and health promotion and disease prevention. He has served as a member of the U.S. Preventive Services Task Force appointed by the assistant secretary for health and is a past president of both the Association for Health Services Research and Foundation for Health Services Research. He is the cofounder of Partnership for Prevention, a coalition of private-sector business and industry organizations that have joined leading health sector organizations in working toward elevating prevention among the nation's health policy priorities. DeFriese is the past editor of *Health Services Research,* the official journal of the Association for Health Services Research, and oversees the Sheps Center's national evaluation of The Robert Wood Johnson Foundation's All Kids Count Childhood Immunization Initiative.

Kathleen M. Faherty, M.S., is a research associate with the Cecil G. Sheps Center for Health Services Research of the University of North Carolina at Chapel Hill, where she is project coordinator for the All Kids Count National Program Evaluation. Prior to coming to the Sheps Center, she served for thirteen years in administrative roles with the North Carolina Area Health Education Centers Program of the University of North Carolina at Chapel Hill School of Medicine. A graduate of Colorado State University and the University of Tennessee, she began her professional career in the education of the hearing impaired and was associated with public school and college teacher preparatory programs.

Victoria A. Freeman, R.N., Dr.P.H., received an undergraduate degree from the University of New Mexico, a nursing degree from the University of Albuquerque, and master's and doctoral degrees in maternal and child health from the school of public health at the University of North Carolina at Chapel Hill. Before pursuing a career in health services research, she served as nurse coordinator with the University of New Mexico Pediatric Oncology Program. She currently works in the area of immunization services research with emphasis on physician behavior, parental knowledge and attitudes, and health care system barriers and enhancements to the receipt of immunization services. Other research interests include the health care needs and services used by children of working women.

Mark A. Goldberg is a distinguished fellow at the Yale School of Management, where he teaches health care policy, political analysis, and nonprofit management. He is also a senior fellow at the Carnegie Foundation for the Advancement of Teaching. He was previously the Lester Crown Visiting Professor of Management at Yale, deputy executive director of the National Leadership Coalition for Health Care Reform, publisher of *The McKinsey Quarterly* as well as director of public affairs at McKinsey & Co., and editor and publisher of *The Brookings Review* at the Brookings Institution. He was a member of the White House staff during the Carter administration, specializing in regulatory and consumer issues. He founded and was editor-in-chief of the *Yale Journal on Regulation* and *Domestic Affairs,* and was cofounder of the Climate Institute. His articles have appeared in a number of publications, including *The New England Journal of Medicine, Health Affairs, The Yale Law Journal, The Washington Post,* and *The Wall Street Journal.*

Priscilla A. Guild, M.S.P.H., has worked in the Cecil G. Sheps Center for Health Services Research at the University of North Carolina at Chapel Hill (UNC-CH) since 1971 and has been deputy director for administrative operations since 1987. In addition, she is adjunct assistant professor in the departments of biostatistics and maternal and child health in the UNC-CH school of public health. Her personal research interests are in the area of health services evaluation, especially as it pertains to primary health care, maternal and child health, and health promotion and disease prevention. For the past twenty years, she has been heavily involved in developing information systems and training related to planning and evaluation for maternal and child health programs at the state and national levels.

Marjorie Gutman, Ph.D., is a senior program officer at The Robert Wood Johnson Foundation. Her responsibilities include overseeing research and program evaluation grants as well as developing new initiatives, primarily in the areas of substance abuse and maternal-child and adolescent health. Prior to coming to the Foundation in 1989, she conducted applied psychological research on reproductive and adolescent health for several years at the Department of Obstetrics and Gynecology, Health Science Center at Brooklyn, State University of New York, and then served as a consultant on maternal-child health to the New Jersey Department of Health.

Julia S. Howard, M.A., is deputy director of The Robert Wood Johnson Foundation Improving Malpractice Prevention and Compensation Systems (IMPACS) program. She previously served as a consultant to the Women's National Breast Cancer Study at the Georgetown University School of Nursing and as a research associate at the Georgetown

University Institute for Health Care Research and Policy. She received her M.A. from the George Washington University School of Government and Business Administration.

Marc S. Kaplan is senior communications officer for The Robert Wood Johnson Foundation. His projects to engage and educate the media through seminars, news media, and special publications have focused on such health care issues as managed care, substance abuse, and care for people with chronic illness and disabilities. Prior to joining the Foundation, he was director for public information for the Rockefeller University in New York City.

Joanne Lynn, M.D., M.A., M.S., is a professor of health care sciences and medicine and the director of the Center to Improve Care of the Dying, a multidisciplinary center committed to research, education, and advocacy to improve the care of seriously ill persons, at the George Washington University Medical Center. She was assistant director of the President's Commission for the Study of Ethical Problems in Medicine and Biomedical and Behavioral Research and codirector of the Study to Understand Prognoses and Preferences for Outcomes and Risks of Treatments (SUPPORT). She has served on the American Bar Association's Commission on Legal Problems of the Elderly, the Board of the American Geriatrics Society, and the Hastings Center Task Force that wrote *Guidelines for the Termination of Treatment and the Care of the Dying*. Lynn was elected to membership in the Institute of Medicine in 1996.

Robert T. Michael, Ph.D., is the Eliakim Hastings Moore Distinguished Service Professor in the Irving B. Harris Graduate School of Public Policy Studies of the University of Chicago. He is also the deputy director of the Northwestern University/University of Chicago Joint Center for Poverty Research. He recently chaired the National Academy of Science/National Research Council Panel on Poverty and Family Assistance. In the area of family economics, Michael has written on the causes of divorce; the reasons for the growth in one-person households; the impact of inflation on families; and the consequences, for the family and especially children, of the rise in women's employment. From 1989 to 1994, Michael served as dean of the Harris School. Earlier, he directed the National Opinion Research Center (NORC) and the West Coast office of the National Bureau of Economics Research.

He has been at the University of Chicago since 1980, having previously taught economics at Stanford University and the University of California, Los Angeles. He is a member of the Board on Children and Families of the Institute of Medicine-National Research Council. Michael was elected a fellow of the American Association for the Advancement of Science in 1994.

Vincent Mor, Ph.D., is the director of the Center for Gerontology and Health Care Research and professor of medical science in the department of community health at the Brown University School of Medicine. He has been principal investigator of numerous foundation and National Institutes of Health grants and contracts to conduct program evaluations in aging and long-term care, including Medicare funding of hospice, the costs and benefits of day hospital treatment and use of home care services, and a national study of residential care facilities. He was an author of the congressionally mandated Minimum Data Set for Nursing Home Resident Assessment and is currently involved in a national evaluation of its implementation. He received a MERIT award from the National Institute on Aging for his research on nursing home organizational factors related to residents' outcomes. He has published more than 150 peer-reviewed articles and several books and chapters on hospice, physical functioning, and long-term care and cancer treatment patterns among the elderly, as well as on measurement of quality of life in various chronically ill populations.

Delores A. Musselman, B.S., is a research assistant with the Cecil G. Sheps Center for Health Services Research at the University of North Carolina at Chapel Hill, where she is associated with the national evaluation of the All Kids Count Childhood Immunization Initiative of The Robert Wood Johnson Foundation.

Debra J. Rog, Ph.D., is a research fellow with the Vanderbilt University Institute for Public Policy Studies and directs the Washington office of the Institute's Center for Mental Health Policy. She is currently the principal investigator of several evaluation and research projects involving systems of health care delivery and services-enriched housing for a variety of populations, including homeless families, families with children in foster care, and single individuals with disabilities. She also directs an evaluation of a funding collaborative of national foundations and federal agencies focused on violence prevention.

Prior to joining Vanderbilt, Rog served as the associate director in the National Institute of Mental Health Office of Programs for the Homeless Mentally Ill. She also worked as a research methodologist for the State of Virginia's Joint Legislative Audit and Review Commission. Rog has published numerous papers on her homelessness research and is a recognized research methodologist, with publications and papers in the areas of applied social research and program evaluation. In addition, she has served as coeditor of the Applied Social Research Methods Series since its inception in 1984, is a coauthor of a text on applied research design, and is the coeditor of a forthcoming *Handbook of Applied Social Research.*

Kristin Nicholson Saarlas, M.P.H., is the assistant deputy director for the All Kids Count Program at the Task Force for Child Survival and Development. Before coming to the task force in 1994, she worked for three years at the Centers for Disease Control and Prevention in the International Health Program Office on malaria control in Africa. Saarlas was a Peace Corps volunteer in Benin, Africa, from 1986 to 1989 in community health and guinea worm eradication and received her master's in public health from Tulane University in 1990.

Lewis G. Sandy, M.D., is executive vice president of The Robert Wood Johnson Foundation. An internist and former health center medical director at the Harvard Community Health Plan, an HMO in Boston, he is also a former Robert Wood Johnson Foundation Clinical Scholar and clinical fellow in medicine at the University of California, San Francisco. Sandy received his M.D. degree from the University of Michigan and his M.B.A. degree from Stanford University. He served his internship and residency at the Beth Israel Hospital in Boston. His activities at the Foundation include working to improve systems of care for people with chronic illness; finding opportunities to help the nation address the problem of escalating medical care costs; and addressing issues of physician supply, distribution, and specialty mix. In addition, he continues to practice and teach at the Robert Wood Johnson Medical School, where he is an assistant clinical professor of medicine.

Steven A. Schroeder, M.D., graduated with honors from Stanford University and Harvard Medical School. He was trained in internal medicine at the Harvard Medical Service of Boston City Hospital, in epidemiology as a member of the Epidemic Intelligence Service of the Communicable Diseases Center (now the Centers for Disease Control and Prevention), and in public health at the Harvard Center for Community Health and Medicine. He served as instructor in medicine at Harvard, assistant and associate professor of medicine and health care sciences at the George Washington University, and associate professor and professor of medicine at the University of California, San Francisco. Since 1990, he has been president of The Robert Wood Johnson Foundation in Princeton, New Jersey, the nation's largest health care philanthropy. He continues to practice general internal medicine on a part-time basis at the Robert Wood Johnson Medical School, where he is clinical professor of medicine. He chairs the international advisory committee of the Faculty of Medicine at Ben-Gurion University in Israel. He has more than 175 publications in the fields of clinical medicine, health care organization and financing, manpower, quality of care, and preventive medicine. From 1987 to 1993, he served as senior editor of the annually updated clinical textbook *Current Medical Diagnosis and Treatment.* He has served on a number of editorial boards, including at present *The New England Journal of Medicine.*

Claudia L. Schur, Ph.D., is deputy director of the Project HOPE Center for Health Affairs. She received her doctorate in economics from the University of Maryland. Her primary areas of interest are health care financing, access and medical care use, and survey design. In addition to her work on the Access-to-Care Survey, Schur is coprincipal investigator on a study of the use of health care services by undocumented immigrants and is working on a study of how managed care organizations manage primary care physicians in prescribing pharmaceuticals, making referrals to specialists, and ordering specific diagnostic and screening tests. Before coming to the Center for Health Affairs, she was at the Agency for Health Care Policy and Research, where she worked on the 1987 National Medical Expenditure Survey. She has published on public and private health insurance coverage for vulnerable populations and the determinants of health care use.

Beth A. Stevens, Ph.D., is a senior program officer at The Robert Wood Johnson Foundation, where she is responsible for research and evaluation in the areas of health care workforce, organization of health care delivery for chronically ill people, and access to health care. Prior to that, she was on the faculty of sociology at New York University, where she did research and taught in the areas of medical sociology and social welfare policy. She received her doctorate in sociology from Harvard University.

Walter Wadlington, L.L.B., is James Madison Professor of Law in the law school and professor of legal medicine in the medical school of the University of Virginia. A member of the American Law Institute and the Institute of Medicine of the National Academy of Sciences, he teaches courses in children's health care, family law, law and medicine, and medical malpractice. He was program director of The Robert Wood Johnson Foundation's Medical Malpractice Program and currently chairs the National Advisory Committee for the Foundation's program on Improving Malpractice Prevention and Compensation Systems. He also serves on the national advisory committee for The Robert Wood Johnson Foundation Clinical Scholars Program.

William C. Watson, Jr., M.P.A., was with the Centers for Disease Control and Prevention for thirty years and was deputy director for twelve years until his retirement in 1984. He was director of operations for the Carter Presidential Center from its opening in 1986 until 1992. He has been associate executive director of the Task Force for Child Survival and Development since its inception in 1984 and is the deputy director of All Kids Count.

Irene M. Wielawski is a freelance journalist who specializes in health care issues. She has written extensively on problems of access to care among the poor and uninsured, and other socioeconomic issues in American medicine. Before taking on the evaluation of The Robert Wood Johnson Foundation's Reach Out program, she was a staff writer and member of the investigations team of the *Los Angeles Times*.

━⁓━ Index

A

Access to care, xi, xiii; and fear of malpractice claims, 118; framework for studying, 58–59; and health care workforce, 23; lack of information on, 55; measuring, 59, 64–65, 70–71; physician volunteer program to increase, 1–20; programs to improve, 83–84; trends in, 73–75

Access-to-care surveys: data collection for, 66; and definitions of financial barriers, 69–70; fine-tuning vs. continuity dilemma for, 68–69; future, 75–76; and health care delivery reform, 71–72; and measuring access, 59, 64–65, 70–71; measuring behavior vs. opinions in, 66–68; national, 55–58; overview of Foundation, 60–63; trends revealed by, 73–75

ACEs (accelerated compensable events), 121

Activities of daily living (ADLs), 140–141

Aday, L. A., 58, 64

Advance directives, by dying patients, 173–174

African Americans: with disabilities, 145; faculty development at colleges for, 31; gonorrhea rate for, 241

Age effect, 240

AIDS: Sexual Behavior and Intravenous Drug Use (National Research Council), 234–235

AIDS: and change in sexual behavior, 244, 247; and need for information on sexual behavior, 234–235

Aiken, L. H., 55

All Kids Count Childhood Immunization Initiative, 189, 192–206; defining immunization registry systems for, 194–195, 196; future of, 205–206; and legislative mandates, 198; overview of, 192–193; public/private sector collaboration in, 199–200; security and confidentiality in, 203–204; size and scope of, 204–205; sponsorship and infrastructure for, 195, 197–198; technology for, 200–203

Alpha Center, 88, 90, 100

Alternative dispute resolution (ADR), for malpractice claims, 120, 128

Alternative medicine, 74

Alternatives to Institutional Maintenance (AIM), 155–156

American Association of Health Plans, Childhood Immunization Practices Survey, 200

American Foundation for AIDS Research, 237

Americans with Disabilities Act (ADA), 134, 144, 157

Andersen, R., 58, 64

Andrew Mellon Foundation, 237

Annie E. Casey Foundation, 193

APACHE II, 170

Association of American Medical Colleges (AAMC), 37

Atkins, T., 19

B

Barone, B. M., 7

Beshear, R., 6, 7

Broadcast journalists, health care reform briefings for, 105–107

Brochure effect, 36

Brown University, disabled population study of, 136

C

California Wellness Foundation, 193

Cardiopulmonary resuscitation (CPR), on dying patients, 168–169, 179

Carnegie Corporation, 28

Case management, 7; for homeless families, 222, 224–226, 227

Catheterization, right heart, 162, 181

Center for Studying Health System Change, 76, 100, 101, 102

Centers for Disease Control (CDC): on AIDS, 234, 235; National Immunization Program (CDC/NIP), 189–190, 195, 206

Certified nurse midwives, workforce programs for, 34, 36, 51